Live Well, Die Happy

Live Well, Die Happy

The Secret Formula for Maximizing
Happiness, Savoring Time, and
Discovering Your Life's Purpose

Eric Metcalf, MPH

RODALE.

© 2017 by Rodale Inc.

Printed in the United States of America

Rodale Inc. makes every effort to use acid-free ∞, recycled paper ♻.

Book design by Carol Angstadt

Library of Congress Cataloging-in-Publication Data is on file with the publisher.

ISBN 978-1-62336-908-8

2 4 6 8 10 9 7 5 3 1 hardcover

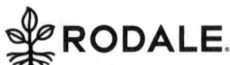

RODALE.

We inspire health, healing, happiness, and love in the world.
Starting with you.

To my family, those who have lived with purpose;
showed grace during adversity; and met the end serenely.
To the ones here now and those who
will ripple us forward.

CONTENTS

Part 4
NOW, ON TO THAT "DYING HAPPY" PART

ACKNOWLEDGMENTS

After my phone conversation with Rodale's editorial director, Anne Egan, I sat in my quiet office contemplating. And perhaps growing a little skeptical.

We had discussed an idea for a possible book that explored death and dying. I agreed that it was an important topic. But now, I wondered, what is there to *say* about death, aside from the core advice: It's no good. Avoid it when possible.

Also, who would *buy* a book about dying? There's no happiness at the end of the discussion. You can't put an encouraging spin on it. You can't land it on a positive note at the last moment. It ends in death.

Was *that* my main kernel of discomfort with this idea? I've been writing consumer health content for 20 years, with some dabbling in health education and healthcare marketing. A book on death seemed to challenge some basic rules I've always followed:

- Point out the barriers that keep readers from living a healthier, happier life . . . then give solutions that move them past these barriers.

- Be ceaselessly positive and focus on the things the reader *can* do. They can take steps to lower their risk of chronic disease—of high blood pressure, of diabetes, of heart disease—and if they do develop one of these, they can find ways to live better with the ailment.

- Give lots of handy tips in bullet points, in lists of three or more.

But a discussion on death whisks you right past all the preventive strategies, right? It acknowledges that someday your pursuit of healthy living will fail.

That said, I do enjoy a challenge. And I've spent too much of my time struggling with life-and-death matters. What am I doing with my life? What would I do if death came for my loved ones? If I'm going to be pondering it anyway, perhaps some good could come of it. So I went to work and started calling the experts.

What I learned was this: No one is really teaching us how to live well, die happy, and tie the two together.

You can find guidance on how to create your will, how to find some peace of mind when you're at the very end, and how to grieve after others have died. I saw lots of very useful bits and pieces, but nothing that seemed to tell the complete story.

There's a great hunger in this country for more openness about What It All Means. It's on the minds of Baby Boomers these days now that they've ticked through many of life's big milestones (kids, career, empty nest, grandkids, retirement) and the big one at the end is looming larger on the windshield.

Death is shedding its taboo status. It's the subject of art festivals across the country. People are gathering to enjoy coffee and wide-ranging discussions about dying. This national conversation is less mournful and more lively than you might expect.

That's the secret I found as I was writing this book. When you think about death, you shouldn't focus on the final moment. Instead think about all that space that carries you from right now to the end.

Then you fill all those moments with life.

Be alive while you're living. If you do it right, the end isn't such a terrible loss.

The terrible loss is not using the rest of your time well.

Over the course of writing this book, I talked to 50-plus people with incredible insight into the death that will come for us, and the life we can strive to achieve before then. Thank you, thank you for sharing your time with me. The ideas that came out of these conversations wove themselves effortlessly into the narrative that runs through this book.

Thanks also to oncologist Larry Cripe, MD, for introducing me to both Terror Management Theory and *The Death of Ivan Ilyich*; and Pastor David Hewitt of the King of Glory church in Carmel, Indiana, for his conversations—particularly the notion that all of us still have something to offer at the very end, no matter how tired or sick we are, even if it's to provide someone else the opportunity to give and to help.

I'm also grateful to the crew at Rodale for coming up with the seed of this book, including Anne Egan and VP Adam Campbell; and to everyone who tightened it up, took out the jokes that went too far, made it look good, and kept me on schedule, including Alisa Bowman, Shea Zukowski, Amy Kovalski, Rana Bumbardatore, Marilyn Hauptly, and Carol Angstadt.

Credit also goes to Brie, my first reader, who continually brings so much good to my life. Let's not let death part us anytime soon, shall we? To my parents, Earl and Marcia, who fueled my early love of words. And, of course, to Ellie, Milo, and Rak. May we all live well together.

INTRODUCTION

Death's Lessons Are Available to All but Heard by Only Some

If you wanted a word to describe this part of central Indiana about 30 miles north of Indianapolis (aside from *flat,* which it very much is), then *orderly* would be a reasonable choice. Country roads crisscross each other at precise 90-degree angles, dividing the landscape into rows of neat squares and rectangles that repeat to the horizon.

The colors across this landscape change predictably, too. The varied shades of soybean and cornstalk green in the summer will yield to the brown of empty, harvested fields when winter returns.

In one of these squares you'll find a spacious, solidly built farm home at the end of a tree-lined drive. This is where Lori Tragesser and her husband, Ben, are raising their five kids.

Sometimes, late at night, Tragesser is the only one awake, struggling with her thoughts. They're some of the most important she's explored in her 45 years.

"When I was first diagnosed, I had all this racing through my head, like thinking about things I want to do with my family, then all of a sudden I'm thinking, 'What will my funeral look like?' or 'Oh, I want to leave *this* for the kids,' or 'I need to sign this.' It's all overwhelming."[1]

So she bought a black notebook and began downloading her biggest worries and fears, drawing them out of her mind and placing them elsewhere so she could rest. "If I thought of something in the middle of the night, I'd remember, 'It's already in the book, I've already written it down.'"

The brush with breast cancer that interrupted Tragesser's regularly scheduled plans will appear like a plot twist in many people's life stories.

In 2016, about 247,000 cases of invasive breast cancer were diagnosed in American women. At some point during their lives, roughly 1 in 8 women born today will develop this disease. Men get it, too, though their lifetime odds are much lower: 1 in 1,000.[2, 3, 4]

So, your story might someday take a turn like Tragesser's did. Mine might, too. It could happen to any of us. The mind-set you'll apply and the strategies you'll use when a life-changing challenge arises will help determine whether you'll continue to live well. In the coming pages, you'll learn how to develop that sort of mind-set and discover those tools.

I'm about 2 years younger than Tragesser. According to a calculator at the Social Security Web site, I can expect to live 13,833 more days if everything works out on average. I seem to have quite a bit more time left—nearly as much as I've spent so far, which has felt like a long time. But those days keep counting down swiftly and steadily.

What will the next one bring? Will I be ready for whatever happens? For Tragesser, quite a few of her days have brought new challenges in recent years.

A radiologist found the grape-size tumor in Tragesser's breast in August of 2012. The cancer was dotted with receptors that allowed it to better absorb fuel for growth. This was actually *good* news. It meant that Tragesser's doctors would have more options to fight the disease.

Tragesser immediately enrolled in a clinical trial and began receiving a drug to block these receptors and hopefully starve the tumor. After just a week, the invader had shrunk to the size of a pea. She then endured 12 treatments of chemotherapy, followed by a double mastectomy the next spring.

Soon, Tragesser was reporting optimistic news on a blog that she updated occasionally for friends and loved ones. She posted pictures from a 5K breast cancer fund-raising race with friends. She shared her hard-won thoughts on how to live not just as a cancer survivor, but a sur*thriver.*[5]

A year after her diagnosis, Tragesser took to her blog to count her blessings. She listed a stronger appreciation for her husband and friends and a new sense of gratitude for her life. She realized that this brush with mortality could have been worse. And she came away from this experience with brand-new, surgically reconstructed breasts.

Then she mostly went quiet, focusing on her job, her family, and her community.

But after another year, Tragesser checked in again, with very different news.

Neither a new pillow nor heat nor massage could resolve the neck pain that kept her from sleeping. A trip to the doctor led to a new round of tests, which brought another diagnosis.

The cancer was back.

This time, it had burrowed into her breastbone. In medical terms, it was now *metastatic* breast cancer. This time, the disease could not be cured. Tragesser will need chemo for the rest of her life to try to control the cancer as well as possible.

Again, Tragesser is not alone here. This event is going to show up in many people's storylines. In 20 to 30 percent of women who have early breast cancer, the disease eventually returns—sometimes quickly, sometimes after decades of silence—and spreads to other parts of the body, such as the bones, brain, liver, or lungs.[6]

"At first, all I could think was, 'I have an average of 3 years to live. What do I need to get done in 3 years?' It was just kind of a panic. I couldn't get anything done because I was trying to deal with this news," she told me.

When Tragesser and I first spoke, she was nearly 2 years into those 3 she had been anticipating.

However, "Somewhere a few months in, I woke up and thought, 'You're only going to live 3 years if that's what you believe you're going to have. You need to change your thinking immediately!' When we built our house, we'd say, 'We'll have *these* bedrooms for the grandkids.' And so I decided to make that my goal, to live to see my grandchildren. That would make it a 10-year plan, rather than 3 years. That's when I got a much better grip."

In this, too, Tragesser is like every single one of us: Right now, she's alive. Someday, she will die. But she truly has no idea when.

It could be next week. On the other hand, doctors reporting in the *Breast Journal* discussed the case of a woman who died in her nineties after living with breast cancer that was in its metastatic form for more than 25 years.[7] So maybe Tragesser's final day will come decades from now. Maybe she'll die of something unrelated to her current condition. Maybe she'll outlive you and me.

In the meantime, Tragesser is spending her time in a way that many of us aren't doing, but should be.

She's living her life deliberately. When a meaningful conversation that she needs to have with one of her kids occurs to her, she jots it down in her black notebook so she'll remember to initiate it at the right moment. She's assembling photo albums of family vacations that have taken them to 41 states and counting. She volunteers in her community, helping to gather back-to-school gear for needy kids in August and Christmas gifts in December. She's active in breast cancer advocacy organizations, and she still works part-time.

Now that she's living more deliberately, she's also considering how she would like her life's end to play out.

"Ben and I bought our plots at the cemetery. When we went, it was like we were picking a lot to build a house on. The Catholic cemetery abuts the golf course, and I said, 'If we were on the back row, we could watch golf all the time, but it's full,' and he joked, 'Well, we don't want to be over here by this tree stump.' In the end, it wasn't a big deal."

She's also been sharing a document called Five Wishes with her friends and family. It's a fill-in-the-blanks tool that guides you to consider five crucial factors that could help determine whether you'll have a so-called good death or whether you'll live your final days under the shadow of indecision, distress, and missed opportunities. (We'll discuss those five factors later in the book.)

"Not long after I was diagnosed, there were two women—both mothers— who died in car crashes in my county. Before their accidents, I'd wondered whether it would be easier to die in a car crash because then you don't have to worry about this stuff or figure it out," Tragesser says. "Then these two ladies died, and I realized, 'I didn't mean that, God! There's so much I can say and do and plan, and that's so much more important than I realized!'

"Just having these end-of-life conversations makes everyone feel better. I think my husband feels better now that we've talked about some of this. I think answering those questions and having those conversations with your children or spouse or parents helps everybody. Then they feel a little more relieved."

Here is where too many of us *haven't* been living like Tragesser.

She's planning how she'd like to navigate the end of her life. She's talking about it with her family, even though that means pushing past the barriers that people build to protect themselves from thoughts of death.

These conversations don't come naturally to everyone. Denying that death awaits us can be easier than accepting it. But today, more people are venturing out of their comfort zones to have these talks, long before a crisis makes it necessary.

They're realizing that they shouldn't wait until they have a serious disease to acknowledge that they'll die someday. They see that their mortality can help propel them through a better life, with more opportunities and richer relationships.

A new way to live well and die happy is spreading. But to access the full benefit of this message, you have to hear it and act on it *now*. If you wait until later, it could be too late.

The realization that you are mortal holds incredible power to change not just the end of your life, but your whole life! Why should you shun death? Why not invite it into your home and offer it a cup of coffee? Death has a message for you. Why not listen to it while you still have years, or even decades, for its wisdom to enrich your life?

Appreciate the Advice That Death Is Trying to Give You

I *may* have an average of 13,833 days remaining, but I also see frequent reminders that I might not make it to the average.

Recently, a father in my community checked in on social media from an annual school fund-raiser event. As the festivities began, he shared a few words of excitement and two photos.

It was his last status update. A few minutes later, he had a fatal heart attack.

The newspaper story revealed that he was my age. In his picture he seemed healthy, and about my size. As far as I could tell, his story and mine had plenty of similarities until that day.

Then came the enlightenment that may occur at these times: "I should enjoy my life more!" I told myself. "I need to be more patient with my kids, less petty with my wife, and less anxious about my deadlines. I *really* need to find my life's passion."

Every week, 50,000 Americans die. When one of them is your coworker, neighbor, or family member, does this moment make you question what you're doing with your life? Does it make you reevaluate how you'd like to spend the time that this person will no longer have?[8]

For readers who were born in 1960, when you were 50 years old, roughly 9 percent of those who shared your birth year had already died from illness or injury. By the time you're 65, that figure will double. When you hear of these losses at your next class reunion, will it give you a flash of gratitude that you're still enjoying life with your loved ones?[9]

If it does, that's great. You're appreciating one of the gifts that mortality offers us. But how long will this wake-up alarm work? If you're like me, you'll hit the snooze button after a few days, or a few weeks at most. Then you'll return to your usual routine of worries, irritations, and streaming TV, interspersed with too few moments of deep-to-your-core *joy*.

The purpose of *Live Well, Die Happy* is to extend that period of wakefulness across more of your days.

When you cultivate a new awareness of how you're spending your life, you can seize opportunities for meaning and growth that otherwise may be overlooked. Because you're making them now—not later—your positive changes have more time to accumulate benefits, like compound interest on each dollar you deposit into a 401(k).

I realize that contemplating your death may seem depressing. The idea that anything good can come from examining such a bleak thought may seem preposterous.

But if you feel like that, perhaps it's because no one has taught you any other way. Generally speaking, America has been a pretty death-averse place in recent generations. Our society has done a good job of shuttling people who are dying into places that are out of view from where the rest of us are living. Thus we can better enjoy our entertainment, our credit cards, and the 360 ads we see each day for products that will make our lives happier.[10]

However, a new willingness to talk about death is blossoming in the United States. The language that people are using to discuss it isn't dour, morose, or despairing. The conversations are breaking out of familiar settings (hospitals and funeral homes) and popping up in more playful venues (art festivals and Twitter).

In the following pages, you'll meet dozens of innovative thinkers who are leading this charge to enliven our discussions about death. Their focus is not just on what death takes from us at the end but also what it can *give* us before then.

You'll also encounter everyday people who ventured closer to death due to illness or accident, then came back from the edge with wisdom that's still influencing their daily thoughts and decisions.

You're about to embark on an exploration. Think of it like a trip to an ancient tomb guarded by a door that may look foreboding at first glance. But inside you'll find valuables that can enrich the rest of your life.

Discover Treasures by Exploring the Idea of Death

Death resists careful examination. On the one hand, it's *huge*. Brilliant people, from ancient philosophers to today's physicians with MRI machines, have spent centuries trying to understand it. A university's worth of theologians, psychologists, and thanatologists couldn't fully explain what it means to die. How far into it could the rest of us expect to get?

dic·tio·nary

Thanatology

The study of death and how we cope with it.

On the other hand, death is *simple* to explain. One moment you're living, the next you're gone. It's so easy, every single person on this planet will eventually do it. You can buy a 99-cent greeting card that sums up death in the most clichéd poetry imaginable. It's coming for all of us, and until then we pay taxes. (That's one of the most common clichés.)

So what's the point in looking more closely at death?

The point is this: With only a minor amount of effort, you can come away with spectacular insight that helps you pack your life with newfound opportunities until it's running over. The lessons that death can teach you are easy to understand today and rich enough to provide ongoing, long-term benefits.

When you open the door to a discussion about death, you'll find the following eight valuables.

1. You can handle the idea of dying. Do you turn away from thoughts about death so they don't grow into a dark cloud that fills your vision? You're going to learn to see your eventual death like a helpful air-traffic controller on the horizon, signaling you to shift your course in a direction that reroutes you through a better life.

Does the concept of death feel like a heavy burden on your shoulders? It doesn't have to be so weighty. You'll meet people who will show you how to carry the right amount of it in your awareness, so it's like a good-luck charm in your pocket that you regularly brush with your fingertips. ("Oh right! *That's* not how I want to be using my precious time. Thanks for the reminder, Death!")

2. Death is steadily influencing you already. Many of the daily choices we make either suppress our awareness that we're going to die or soothe us when this knowledge leaks into our consciousness. A well-researched area of psychology has found that we assemble many of the factors that make us who we are—our preferences, our hobbies, our friends, our identity—to cope with the fear of death. But we don't often realize we're doing it. (We'll explore this concept more in Chapter 1.)

Death is already a powerful motivator in your life. But it doesn't always propel you where you really want to go. If that engine is going to be moving you anyway, wouldn't you be better off steering it with more control?

3. You can reverse-engineer a better life by looking to the end. For many people, the end of life is a time of important reflection. What did they do that brought happiness? What choices led to regret and guilt? What unfinished business still needs to be squared away? Hospice professionals, palliative care doctors, and clergy witness this reflection, and they'll share with you the factors that are often on people's minds at the end of life.

You can use this knowledge like a map. If you sense that *this* will be a source of comfort in your final months or *that* is likely to be a source of suffering, you can make choices now that will lead you to a more peaceful and satisfying conclusion.

4. Living well requires a balance between dedication and flexibility. A well-lived life requires deliberate planning. To achieve it, you need goals and the willpower to achieve them. However, the world will continually try to redirect you. Your health will change. Your surroundings will shift. Familiar people will exit your life, and new ones will enter.

It's important to keep moving toward a destination on the horizon while staying nimble enough to shift to a new path if necessary. If you stick to a course that you no longer have the resources to follow, or you demand results that you can't attain, you set the stage for an unhappy life.

5. To die well, practice "learning to live with loss." Dan Moseley, DMin, a retired pastor, author, and widower, shared this powerful idea with me outside a Starbucks one sunny morning. How well you cope with loss is also going to be a major determinant in how much meaning and happiness you find in your life.[11]

We're *continually* facing losses over the course of our lives, Dr. Moseley says. Some losses we feel immediately, and some only break into our awareness over time. Our childhood ends. The customs of our youth are thrown out by the next generation. The face in the mirror turns into a different face. We lose an athletic ability. Loved ones die. We change jobs, and later we retire. Each of these losses is like the death of a little part of our existence, he says. On one of our future days, we will face the biggest loss, which is the loss of life.

You don't have to love these little "practice deaths" that will occur. But you do need to cope with them, learn from them, and fit them into the fuller story of your life. By doing so, your own death may become easier to accept.

6. You must do it now. Later may not arrive. For most of us, the situation that could cause our eventual death will give us advance notice. We may use this time like Lori Tragesser has been doing in recent years: taking care of unfinished business, having important conversations, and making end-of-life plans.

On the other hand, some of us will die suddenly. Maybe you'll clutch your head and be gone. Or maybe you'll be hit by a bus. (This is another common death cliché, but it's quite unlikely. In 2013, only 64 pedestrians in America died this way.)[12]

If your death is sudden, you likely won't have time to address unfinished business. (Or if you slip into a fog of dementia before you die, it will be too late for any actions you want to take or words you want to say.)

You're going to learn a lot of strategies for living well and dying happy. As I'll keep saying, the best practice is to do them *now*. "Now" is a moment you know you have. "Later" is not.

7. Every bit of your life counts. The end of your life presents opportunities for incredible growth. Your final days aren't just the few unusable pennies you have left from your dollar or the last drops of soda that you don't bother trying to slurp out of the can.

Though the end of your life may not prompt you to make a Hollywood-style tearjerker of a speech, this time has the potential to stand alongside the momentous days that marked your graduation, your wedding, or the birth of a child. In these days, you can repair relationships, edit your legacy, share unforgettable words, and give your loved ones assistance that may help them through their grief.

But we can trace your important days back further.

Even the time you spend struggling with the symptoms of a chronic illness is valuable. So are the days you spend struggling with loss. Whether you're operating at the peak of your powers or you're capable only of voicing a few well-chosen words, *all* your time matters, from now to the end. It's *all* worth using as well as you can.

8. You're not the only one who decides whether your life was lived well. Right now, you're the central figure in determining whether your beliefs and your actions add up to a happy and meaningful life. But as soon as you're gone, the people around you—your community, friends, coworkers, and loved ones—will have the last word.

If the central passion that drives the brief time you're alive is your career or your investment accounts, will those who shared your life remember you as a full, complete person? Or will they speak of you fondly while thinking to themselves, "Yes, but . . . "?

While reading this book, you'll learn how to create a well-balanced life that both rewards you and provides dividends for the people who remain after you're gone.

When we last spoke, new spots of cancer had appeared in Tragesser's ribs, and her fourth type of chemotherapy was causing side effects that sounded quite unpleasant. Yet her voice was cheerful as she steered the conversation to one of her kids' soccer success. "The facts of my disease and my future are extremely unsettling, yet there is no other way to live," she wrote in her blog. "Living with a terminal illness is a continuous process of dealing with what happens in your body next . . . balancing optimism with reality, capturing the beautiful moments of your life, and ultimately choosing to live each day doing what matters to you most."

Tragesser regularly faces reminders that her life will someday end, but she's still finding ways to live well. Now is the best time for the rest of us to figure out how to do this, too.

Before we embark on this exploration, I'd like to note one important issue this book *won't* tackle. For many, the most essential question associated with death is, "What happens to me after I die?" But *Live Well, Die Happy* is not going to try to answer that question. You can examine that topic in plenty of other books, some with thousands of years' worth of dedicated followers.

That said, an important theme of this work is how to find meaning in your life, which for many people involves religious or spiritual practice. *Live Well, Die Happy* recognizes this type of faith, and it includes advice from some experts with insight into it. But if you don't tend to spiritual matters—or you believe that all you'll ever have is right here during your time on Earth—this book will also help you get the most from your life.

The conversation you're about to join is for everyone who's alive and everyone who's going to die. That's you, me, and all the people you'll meet in the coming pages. I think you're going to have fun. This discussion veers into death at times, but when it does, it's a *lively* discussion about death.

Part I

DEATH HAS A MESSAGE FOR YOU

Right now, you're standing at Point A.

Someday—which could come quite soon, or perhaps not for another century, if scientists keep making breakthroughs—you'll reach Point B. That's your final day. A lot of stuff will occur along the line between them. Good stuff, exciting stuff, boring stuff, bad stuff. Who knows what you'll get!

The challenges that the world throws in your path will help determine whether you live well and die happy. But a much bigger deciding factor will be how you *plan* for those challenges and *think* about them when they arise.

You're now holding a guidebook for the adventure you'll have between Point A and Point B. Here's a general map of where the coming sections of the book will take you.

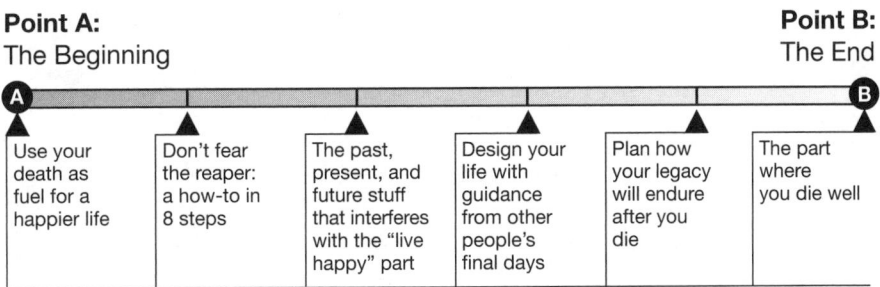

Point A:
The Beginning

Point B:
The End

| Use your death as fuel for a happier life | Don't fear the reaper: a how-to in 8 steps | The past, present, and future stuff that interferes with the "live happy" part | Design your life with guidance from other people's final days | Plan how your legacy will endure after you die | The part where you die well |

Along this route, you'll learn how to reduce your dread of your inevitable death. You'll learn how to better manage the common rough patches that make life more difficult. You'll also give thought to choices that will strengthen the legacy that will carry on after you're gone.

Ultimately, by doing the advance work outlined in this book, you can someday even navigate the end of your life with greater peace of mind.

Use Your Death as Fuel for a Happier Life

When people engage in wishful thinking and denial, they may picture their future years looking a little like this graph:

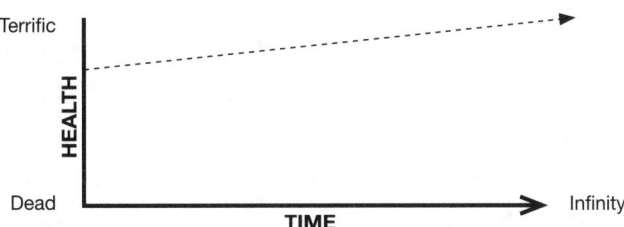

You can interpret this as, "I'm going to live forever, baby! If anything, I'm just going to keep getting better!"

But in reality, our future life and death will likely unfold in one of the following patterns, or *trajectories,* according to the Institute of Medicine.[1]

The least common type is the swift death: the massive heart attack, drowning, or violent event that steals a life with little to no warning. In other words, you're going along fine, then it's over. The vertical axes of the graphs on pages 3 and 4 represent your health, and the horizontal axes represent the length of your life.

The graph above is adapted with permission from the National Academies Press, © 1997, National Academy of Sciences.

3

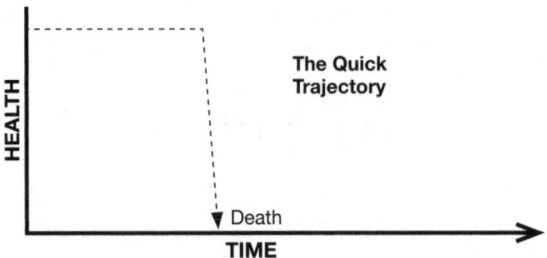

More commonly, your health can steadily decline over a long period of time, then fall off rapidly at the end. Some cases of cancer follow this trajectory. You may also see this with dementia or in old age when your body's internal organs just can't keep functioning.[2]

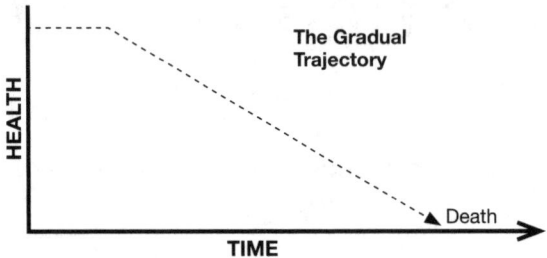

Or you may have a condition that's treatable but that gradually worsens over the years and from time to time causes a health crisis. These emergencies could lead to a trip to the hospital, and one of them could even prove fatal (the vertical lines) if your doctors can't get it under control. Congestive heart failure, in which damage to your heart keeps it from pumping properly, can cause this. So can chronic lung disease, such as COPD.

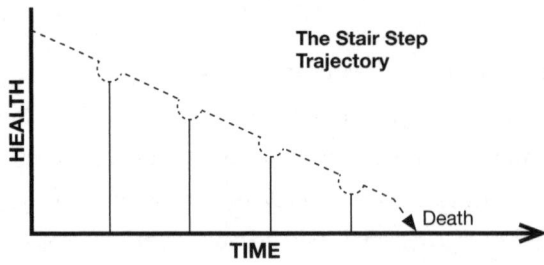

The graphs above are adapted with permission from the National Academies Press, © 1997, National Academy of Sciences.

Clearly, all these trajectories end in the same point. So let's just say what that point is, since it's that kind of book. No matter what sort of story you write for your life, it will end in death. (Spoiler alert—this book will, too!)

Traditionally, death has been a taboo topic in many circles. Such a difficult idea should be couched in euphemisms—you pass away, or perhaps you depart—or better yet, it shouldn't be discussed at all.

But times are changing. If you're not willing to chat about your eventual demise, you might find yourself missing some fun parties. That's because a growing number of people are talking about death, and they're having a good time doing it.

Rather than a morbid and unpleasant task, these conversations may even be a piece of cake, as one recent start-up hoped.

Cake—a tool for self-discovery that was released on a Web site (JoinCake .com)—asks you to consider a series of statements about the end of your life.

- When I am gone, I would want my Facebook profile to be deleted. Agree or disagree?

- I feel at peace with how I've lived my life so far. Agree or disagree?

- I would stay at my job even if I only had 1 year to live. Agree or disagree?

After you ponder enough of these questions, your philosophy about important end-of-life issues begins to take shape. You start to envision the type of life-sustaining medical treatment you might want; how you'd like your life to be remembered when you're gone; whether your legal and financial affairs are in order; and the type of funeral or memorial service you might like. Of course, it's also likely that your responses will highlight knowledge gaps in your end-of-life plans.

This light touch helps people who might otherwise shrink away from doing end-of-life planning because it feels like a difficult slog, says Suelin Chen, PhD, who cofounded the start-up with a palliative care doctor. It also gives your loved ones useful answers to questions that a lawyer probably wouldn't ask, such as what type of foods you'd want at your memorial service or whether you'd like your loved ones to drink to your memory on the anniversary of your death.[3]

Pondering your mortality may lead you to ask yourself other questions that could open your life to more joy, like: *At the end, will I feel that I made a meaningful difference in the world?* If your answer is no, perhaps it's time to live differently!

The Right Questions Can Trigger a Conversation about Life Planning

A group-based conversation game called My Gift of Grace—appeared to coax people to think more about their end-of-life health-care wishes, according to a study presented in 2016 in the *American Journal of Hospice & Palliative Care Medicine*.[4]

Sixty-eight people played the game, considering questions like: "In order to provide the best care possible, what three nonmedical facts should your doctor know about you?" During the following 3 months, 78 percent of the players did some type of advance-care planning behaviors, like sharing end-of-life wishes with loved ones or discussing their thoughts on *quality* versus *quantity* of life.

This type of planning can spark interesting conversations now, and it can make life better for you and your family later. The game is available for order online, but you'll also find similar thought-provoking questions at the end of each chapter in this book.

Death: A Conversation Starter That Brings Young and Old Together

The nation's growing openness about death may be yet another social change that Baby Boomers are propelling, says Harriet Warshaw, the executive director of The Conversation Project. Her organization also creates easy-to-use materials to start you thinking about end-of-life issues and discussing your wishes with your loved ones. (That second step is crucial.)[5]

"There's been a remarkable shift in our culture. When we started 5 years ago, people couldn't utter the words. Now there's more awareness; you can barely read the popular press without seeing something about this topic," she says.

"I do think it is coming from the Boomers, who have experienced end-of-life crises with their parents or loved ones. They're seeing how the system is not people-friendly; it rarely helps identify what matters most to people and how they want to live at the ends of their lives. The Baby Boomers are saying, 'We've changed the way we deliver our babies, and now we want to change the way we die. We want to have more control over it.'"

However, the Boomers aren't the only ones growing more comfortable with discussing death. So are their kids and grandkids.

While I was writing this book, *The Fault in Our Stars,* a love story of two teens with cancer, was celebrating more than 141 weeks on the *New York Times* young adult bestseller list. The subsequent movie adaptation brought in more than $300 million.[6,7]

Social media is turning mortuary insiders into minor celebrities. Caitlin Doughty, a funeral home owner, answers questions on her campy "Ask a Mortician" YouTube channel. Caleb Wilde, a 30-something, sixth-generation funeral director in Pennsylvania, shares deep insight and groan-worthy puns on Twitter and Facebook. (Sample wisdom: "If you found out you were dying, would you be nicer, love more, try something new? Well, you are. We all are.")[8]

In 2011, a series of informal get-togethers called the Death Cafe began in the United Kingdom and soon came to the United States. Its purpose is "to increase awareness of death with a view to helping people make the most of their (finite) lives." At the free-ranging discussions, participants "eat cake, drink tea, and discuss death." Thus far, organizers have hosted more than 3,700 around the world.[9]

However, though more people are answering the question, "Have you prepared for the end of your life?" with *yes,* not everyone's on board yet.

Denial of Death May Leave You Unprepared When You *Have* to Face It

In 2013, only 37 percent of Americans said they'd given "a great deal of thought" to the type of medical treatment they would want at the end of life, according to a Pew Research Center survey. That was just a moderate increase from 28 percent back in 1990. Another 35 percent had given it "some" thought.[10]

Even when they're at a later age, advance care planning still isn't on a lot of people's minds. In 2016, researchers from the University of California, San Francisco, found that more than a quarter of people ages 65 and older hadn't had any discussions or made any plans concerning their end-of-life preferences.[11]

---

dic·tio·nary

Advance directive

This is a legal document that spells out the types of treatments you would want if you were ever unable to speak for yourself during a life-threatening medical situation. Treatments covered include CPR, receiving nutrients through an IV, defibrillation (shocking the heart to get it into a normal rhythm), and use of a ventilator (breathing machine).[12]

Because your wishes will likely change over time it's important for you to not just create an advance directive but also to review it on occasion and update it as necessary. Turn to page 180 for specific details on how to create one.

The idea of preparing for the end of your life may feel uncomfortable for many reasons. Common explanations people give for why they don't want to have these conversations include:

- Simply not wanting to think about dying

- A poor understanding of the healthcare options available at the end of life

- Uneasiness about pulling family or friends into these discussions

You may be surprised to learn that your healthcare providers may also have difficulty discussing end-of-life issues with you for their own reasons. In one 2015 study, nurses and doctors who cared for hospitalized patients noted that the following barriers often prevented these conversations.[13]

- Patients and their family members didn't want to accept that their medical problems could lead to death.

- Patients and families had trouble understanding that life-sustaining medical treatments often have limitations at the end of life and also that they can cause serious complications.

- Family members disagreed about the results they wanted the treatments to provide.

- Patients were simply not in a state to make decisions.

Some physicians don't have any formal training on how to discuss end-of-life care. A busy doctor may not have time to carry out this conversation. She may not want to initiate a talk that might upset you. She may think that if she brings up death, you'll feel that she's "giving up" on you. Or, she may be waiting for *you* to start the conversation.

Odds are good that someday a doctor will need to know what kind of end-of-life medical treatment you want. The answers that you or a loved one provide may help determine whether you have that "die happy" ending.

If you're not ready to accept the idea that you will die someday, now is the time to start shifting your thinking. By planning for your future and having tough-but-necessary family conversations on an ongoing basis, you can better navigate the end of your life on *your* terms. Your choices will more likely match your needs and values.

You may also help your loved ones get through your final days with greater harmony and peace of mind, as well as less conflict and regret.

But if you're in denial that you're going to die someday, you're less likely to do this advance work.

What Your Future Likely Holds at Its End

If you had shopped for a useful book on dying in an earlier era—say around 1900—you might have picked up something like *How to Stay Alive Past 50—Or Even 60!* Or maybe *Why So Many Hearses in My Neighborhood?*

Not long ago, our life expectancy was much shorter. A baby girl born in 1900 had a fifty-fifty shot of reaching her late forties. Males generally died a bit earlier—around age 46, on average. Aside from a brief, sharp drop in 1918 due to a deadly flu pandemic, the subsequent century steadily added decades to our life expectancy.[14, 15]

You probably already knew this. But these familiar numbers carry some interesting details that help explain our national discomfort with dying.

For starters, when death came back then, it typically moved quickly. In 1900, nearly half of Americans died of infections like pneumonia, flu, and digestive illnesses. So people's departures were often swift and jarring, and at an age when they were still very active and visible in their communities.[16]

Also, when our great-great grandparents were near the ends of their lives, they were more likely to stay right where they were. Often, their families cared for them at home in their final days, and they died in their own beds.[17]

But throughout the 1900s, the way we died changed considerably. Death became more drawn out and less visible. The public gained the ability, to some degree, to not have to think about it.

Today, heart disease and cancer alone account for 46 percent of all deaths in the United States. Other causes in the top 10 list include chronic lung disease, stroke, Alzheimer's, diabetes, and kidney disease.[18]

These conditions may cause months, years, or even decades of gradual decline. People can keep working, raising their families, and showing up at social gatherings with problems that may ultimately be fatal. So, many of us seldom see someone who's actively dying, compared to our ancestors' experiences.

Also, when our friends, relatives, and neighbors died in recent decades, they often went somewhere else to do it.

The number of acute-care hospitals in the United States reached a high of 7,200 near the end of the 1900s. With antibiotics, CT scans, and surgeries and other treatments for cancer and other chronic diseases, hospitals can often—but not always—buy even severely ill people more time. In 2000, half of all deaths in the United States occurred in hospitals. Roughly 25 percent more occurred in nursing homes or other long-term care facilities.[19, 20]

Medical providers in hospitals often fight the dying process aggressively rather than managing it as a natural event. One quarter of the money Medicare spends on medical treatments for seniors—which adds up to $125 billion annually—ends up supporting people who are in their final year of life.[21] But ultimately these medications, invasive tests, imaging, and surgical procedures may do relatively little to extend lives, and they can leave patients feeling much *worse* during any extra time they buy at the very end.

In short, today's middle-aged and older adults simply haven't had the same exposure to dying as a normal part of life, compared to our predecessors just a few generations ago. As a publication from the Institute of Medicine noted in 1997, "Adults, even into middle age, may never have lived near or cared for someone who was dying." To quote from another book on death: "A long-distance phone call announcing the passing of grandpa or grandma takes the place of the intimate, firsthand experience of a loved one's death."

If you think that death is largely something that "old" people do, you're correct. If you have never witnessed someone in the final stages of dying, that's not surprising either. In recent times, many people's final days have unfolded in antiseptic rooms in big buildings miles from home.

But just as dying changed radically during the 20th century, the pendulum is now swinging in a new direction. With an immense population of Baby Boomers crossing the finish line in the next 20 years, it's not obvious how we can keep paying for any end-of-life care that doesn't have a clear benefit. And this generation, which is long accustomed to having their say, is now supporting a shift in how we die.

In coming years, you can expect to have growing control over your medical choices at the end of your life. Fewer people are now dying in institutions; in 2014, just 37 percent of people died in a hospital. From 2000 to 2014, the number of people who died at home jumped nearly 30 percent.[22]

If you want to die at home, which surveys indicate is the wish of most Americans, *hospice care* can help you do so more comfortably. In 1982, only 25,000 people used these services at the end of life. By 2014, more than 1.6 million people who were dying looked to hospice providers for care.[23]

In addition, a new branch of medicine called *palliative care* has arisen. It focuses on managing uncomfortable symptoms, including those experienced at the end of life. More than two-thirds of American hospitals with 50 or more beds offered a palliative care team in 2015, compared to just over half in 2008.[24]

dic·tio·nary

Hospice

This is a type of care that's intended to keep you as physically comfortable as possible at the end of life, and it also supports your mental, emotional, and spiritual well-being. Hospice care comes from a team of providers that may include one or more doctors, nurses, social workers, health aides, chaplains, and volunteers. You can receive these services in your home, a hospital, a nursing home, or a hospice facility.[25]

Hospice care is not intended to cure the disease that will likely end your life, and it's typically for people who are expected to live no more than 6 months. But using hospice services doesn't mean you're giving up on life. Research found that people with congestive heart failure or several types of cancer lived an average of 29 days longer with hospice care.[26]

Palliative care

This is a branch of medicine that focuses on relieving symptoms (like pain, nausea, fatigue, and insomnia) rather than curing an underlying disease. Though it's often associated with end-of-life care, palliative care doctors also help people who are seriously ill but not dying, while their other doctors try to manage their disease or injury.

However, before you can use hospice services, you and your loved ones may have to make some tough decisions. You may need to acknowledge that another medication, MRI scan, or surgery is not going to fix you. You may have to shift gears and say, "Okay, this is it. I choose not to deny my death or keep fighting it, but to accept it. I want to spend the remainder of my time doing something else."

In the next chapter, you're going to learn how to develop a new relationship with your death. The goal is to maintain awareness that you'll die and to accept its inevitability. You may still have some fear of death, and it can still make you sad, but this fear and sadness shouldn't paralyze you or interfere with your enjoyment of life.

But proceed with caution: Getting more comfortable with your mortality will require you to adjust your grip on a burden that humanity has been carrying for millennia.

The Dreadful Truth That Propels Us All

Compared to the rest of the animals on this planet, humans have it pretty good. For starters, we get a long life. While as a species our longevity comes nowhere close to some mollusks and giant tortoises that can live hundreds of years, you can expect to have a longer life than most of the animals you see on a daily basis.

We also get to live inside. That's something! Most of us don't wake up every day to another fight for our survival, either. Feeding ourselves is relatively easy when we can choose from a long list of occupations that aren't physically taxing. The opposable thumbs are nice, too.

On the other hand, humans are uniquely unfortunate in one regard: We appear to be the only creatures that know we're going to die. Other animals will desperately fight and flee to stay alive. But they probably can't foresee that one day their effort will fail.

No matter what qualities help you solve your more minor concerns—speed, strength, creativity, smarts, looks, money, or luck—none will help you conquer this final problem. And somewhere inside that computer you call your brain is a line of code that keeps reminding you that you will die.

"This awareness of death is the downside of human intellect. . . . On one hand, we share the intense desire for continued existence common to all living things; on the other, we are smart enough to recognize the ultimate futility of this fundamental quest. We pay a heavy price for being self-conscious," wrote the creators of a psychological concept called the *Terror Management Theory* in their 2015 book, *The Worm at the Core*.[27]

This theory, called TMT for short, asserts that the awareness that we're

What's a "Good Death," Anyway?

I'd like for you to start creating a vision of the sort of end-of-life period you'd like to have someday. Whenever you see the term *good death,* it will refer to that image.

The Institute of Medicine's definition of a good death is one that is "free from avoidable distress and suffering for patients, families, and caregivers; in general accord with patients' and families' wishes; and reasonably consistent with clinical, cultural, and ethical standards."

Not everyone is a fan of this phrase. "I'm a little allergic to the term 'good death.' I think there's this idea that if only I can do all this planning, I can die the way I want to die," says Meredith MacMartin, MD, a palliative care doctor and assistant professor at Dartmouth's Geisel School of Medicine in Hanover, New Hampshire.[28]

Planning for your end is like preparing for the type of childbirth you want, in terms of the control you have over the results, Dr. MacMartin says. You may spend 9 months setting the stage for an at-home birth with a midwife, soft lighting, and your favorite music, but if the power goes out or an unforeseen complication requires you to have an emergency C-section, you will end up delivering in a hospital.

Similarly, not everyone who wants to die at home does so. Some people die unexpectedly while in the hospital. In other cases, their family members can't take care of them at home at the end.

You get to define what a good death means to you. But it's important to realize that you probably won't be fully in control when the time comes. Sufficient planning will go a long way toward helping you achieve your good death. But make room for "good" to encompass unplanned developments.

going to die fuels many feelings and activities that make us human. Frequently, your thoughts and behaviors help you manage this dreadful truth.

According to TMT, a crucial way that we manage our fear of death is to identify with long-standing cultures such as our nation, religion, ethnic background, university, or even professional sports team. Then we do the things that our fellow members within that culture do.

We're here for only a brief time, but the cultural structures that existed before us will likely continue after we leave. By tossing a little bit of ourselves into these sprawling, timeless pools, some part of us lives on after we're gone. We want these institutions to embrace us. We want them to nourish us, and in return to accept the contributions we give them. So we devote our loyalty to them, and we defend them from ridicule and threat.

Another important way we try to extinguish our fear of death is to bolster our self-esteem, which the TMT developers define as "a feeling of personal significance." People measure their personal significance in all manner of ways around the globe: height; bank account balance; strength; number of livestock owned; number of states or countries checked off on the back of the RV.

We participate in our culture and protect our self-esteem every single day. We vote for the candidate who promises to change the nation in ways we find appealing. We join others in pursuing a common goal, whether by playing on a softball league after work or picking up trash along the road on a community volunteering day. We wash our faces and brush our teeth in the morning, and we walk on the treadmill and do situps at night.

But sometimes, we also think and do selfish or unkind things in the pursuit of tamping down our fear of death. For proof, consider the classic study from 1998 that involved several clever researchers and plenty of homemade hot sauce.[29]

The researchers recruited college students who described themselves as moderately conservative or liberal. The students wrote either a detailed description of a scenario in which they died or a nonthreatening scene in which they took an exam. (TMT-related studies typically expose participants to thoughts of death, such as by asking them to envision dying.) Finally, the students read a short essay from a "fellow student" that was either strongly hostile toward liberals or conservatives.

Despite this setup, the students thought they were participating in a taste-testing exercise. The researchers asked them to spoon out a dollop of hot sauce, which the "fellow student" who wrote the essay would eat. It was composed of "5 parts Heinz chili sauce and 3 parts Tapatío salsa picante hot sauce" and was "indeed quite hot."

Among the students who had to imagine their deaths, those who read an essay that ridiculed their political view served up an especially big dose of spicy sauce for the author to eat. According to the researchers, this experiment clearly supported the idea that having death on your mind can make you more aggressive toward people who threaten your worldview.

After all, people who think differently about important issues are implying that our beliefs are incorrect, aren't they? They may even be trying to damage the cultural structures that we want to outlast us! As a result, the researchers suggest that the mortality-related unease at humanity's core could be a substantial driver of violent conflicts around the world.

Since then, other experiments have also found that thoughts about death may make us more likely to:

- Believe more strongly that our romantic partners have good feelings about us[30]
- Want to buy products advertised on television[31]
- Conversely, adopt money-saving habits[32]
- Look negatively upon undocumented immigrants[33]
- Define effective leaders as those with more "masculine" qualities (like being more analytical, ambitious, and competitive rather than supportive, warm, and sensitive to others' needs)[34]
- Want to name our children after ourselves, particularly if we're having higher levels of anxiety[35]

So why is it useful to understand that our relationship with death takes place against this sort of backdrop? There are a few reasons.

Our unconscious feelings about death have power. All sorts of forces that operate below your awareness influence your thoughts and behaviors: events from childhood you don't even remember, messages you've incorporated from the media, your brain chemistry, and so on.

Like the multiple propellers on the drones that fly over our public spaces these days, these forces move you. And the natural dread you feel about death seems to be a particularly insistent source of propulsion.

It's unlikely that you can lose your fear of death completely—and doing so would not be healthy, even if you could. But you should learn to handle your feelings about death so they're less likely to blow you off course.

Your feelings about mortality can make your life better. Or worse. In 2015, a pair of psychologists wrote a paper for the journal *Social Sciences* that offered "an appreciative view of the brighter side of terror management processes."[36]

If physical fitness is a priority, unconscious thoughts of your death may prompt you to work out. If you read messages that a pale complexion is more attractive or that the people around you find smoking repulsive, you may be less likely to visit a tanning parlor or light a cigarette, the authors write. (After all, you don't want your culture to reject you!)

Death thoughts may also prompt you to seek out romantic relationships and stay in them instead of looking for the exit; the authors cite a drop in divorce rates in the Oklahoma City region after its 1995 bombing. Dread of death may also fuel your creativity and spur you to seek adventure.

On the other hand, if you have a large reservoir of death anxiety, it can seep out in ways that reduce your quality of life. Death anxiety may play a role in health anxiety, the excessive preoccupation with the idea that you're currently sick or will fall ill in the future, says Lisa Iverach, PhD, a research fellow at the University of Sydney, Australia. (Health anxiety is another term for hypochondria.) In some people, death anxiety also fuels other types of psychological distress, like depression, eating disorders, social anxiety, obsessive-compulsive disorder, and post-traumatic stress disorder (PTSD).[37]

According to TMT, when death leaks into our conscious awareness (for example, when a classmate or an acquaintance dies), we have a dual response, Dr. Iverach says. One response is conscious: Perhaps we wear our seat belt next time we drive, or we order the medium pizza instead of the large. The other is unconscious: We do things to support our culture or boost our self-esteem without thinking about them.

"When we look at people with anxiety disorders, there's some disruption to that process. They're washing their hands, saying, 'I'm so afraid of germs that could make me sick or make my family sick, what if we die?' It's not necessarily a conscious process, but it leaks out into behaviors," Dr. Iverach says. "Or people who have phobias of spiders, or blood, or heights. All those things are related to death. For vulnerable individuals, that fear of death drives a lot of their anxious behaviors and responses. Anxiety disorders affect 10 percent of the population, so we're actually talking about a large group."

Throughout this book, you're going to have opportunities to assess your emotions, behaviors, and motivations. As you do, see if you can determine how your feelings about death might have prompted you to live a life that's more fearful—and how they might help you create a more courageous, fearless future.

Your thoughts on mortality can make the *world* better. Or worse. In some situations, thinking about your death might encourage you to help others or protect the environment, according to the authors of that "brighter side of terror management" paper.

" . . . It is common for cultural worldview beliefs to promote values and standards of worth that direct people to treat each other, for example, fairly and with compassion. Second, cultivating and contributing to positive social groups is one way to gain a sense of worth and protect the prominence and permanence of one's culture," they write.

On the other hand, many early studies on TMT looked at negative effects, such as prejudice, that are linked to our thoughts on death. These "helped set the stage for a 25-year track record of TMT research demonstrating the impact of death awareness on harmful personal and social consequences," according to the researchers.

Over and over, you're going to read in the following pages that if you want a life of meaning and happiness, you're going to find it in connections with other people. Some of the people you'll encounter will be familiar. They are going to look like you and participate in your culture, and they may include your spouse, kids, coworkers, fellow worshippers, and the bulk of your Facebook friends.

But many of the people you might encounter in person or through the media *won't* be part of your culture. They may make very different choices than you would. They may disagree with some of your beliefs that calm your fears of death.

You can go the rest of your life feeling anger and contempt toward people who are different than you. While you're at it, you can keep drawing the circle that encompasses "people like me" smaller and smaller, until you're just down to yourself. Or you can go big with your brief time on Earth, making a positive impact that reverberates far and wide.

Each of us hears different messages from the death that awaits us. Some of them are clearly negative ("life is ultimately meaningless"). Some might seem correct on their face but can lead us astray ("outsiders are threatening my way of life").

But some messages convey wisdom that we'd better heed. They might emphasize the importance of treating time as a limited resource we can't waste; distributing the best parts of ourselves into the world so they can live on; and staying active, vital, and *alive* for as long as we are living.

"I have friends who said to me when they found out I'm interested in death anxiety, 'Don't even talk to me about it! I'm so terrified of dying or my children dying that I can't even talk about that subject!'" Dr. Iverach told me.

"But I think I'm *glad* I've become involved in this research because it's made me reflect on living a good life so eventually I'll have a good death," she says. "At first, I was a little overwhelmed by how often I was thinking about death. But now—well, *pleasant* may be too lovely a word—but it drives my behavior more in terms of how I think about things, choices I make, and how I respond to people around me."

LIVE WELL, DIE HAPPY EXERCISES
Chapter 1

At the end of each chapter, I'd like you to answer a few questions so that by the end of the book you'll have a better understanding of your death, and the life you'll live before it comes.

The following themes will help you get a baseline sense of your core feelings toward death and dying. Please answer these questions on the lines below or in a separate notebook, if you wish.

1. What experiences have you had with the deaths of loved ones and friends? Do you think they had "good deaths" as defined on page 14? If so, what qualities during their lives do you think influenced their deaths (such as acceptance, curiosity, openness to having tough conversations, or a sense of adventure)? _____

_____

_____

_____

_____

2. How much end-of-life planning (such as writing your will or buying a cemetery plot) have you done? If you haven't done any, what's truly holding you back? (Go beyond "it costs too much" or "it's too much hassle.") _____

_____

_____

_____

_____

3. If your parents are alive, can you talk easily with them about their eventual deaths? Can you talk about your own eventual death with your spouse or kids? If not, why? Are you afraid you'll scare them? Will it force you to discuss other uncomfortable issues about your family? _____

_____

_____

_____

_____

4. How's your physical health? Are you currently living with an illness that could end your life or limit your activities? Does it make you live a smaller life, or does it prompt you to live more fully *despite* the illness? _____

_____

_____

_____

_____

_____

5. How's your mental health? Do you have any depression or anxiety that might be linked to a fear of death, sickness, change, or aging? _____

_____

_____

_____

_____

_____

6. What are the important cultural structures in your life? Do you define yourself by your profession, your nationality, your military service, your religion, or your hobbies? _____

_____

_____

_____

_____

_____

7. If you were to die today, what would the people around you—your spouse, kids, extended family, coworkers, and friends—miss most about you? _____

_____

_____

_____

_____

_____

CHAPTER 2

Pull Off Death's Scary Mask

As she stirred a pot of noodles on the stove, the spoon slipped from Ashlyn Blocker's hand into the boiling water. Instinctively, the Georgia teen reached in, felt around for the spoon, and retrieved it.[1]

She didn't cry out in pain because she didn't feel any. She never has.

It's easy to imagine the benefits of being immune to pain. You'd never know the maddening annoyance of a paper cut. You could enjoy a pleasant trip to the dentist for a root canal. Life inflicts pain on our bodies relentlessly, and to rise above physical discomfort would be a welcome superpower, wouldn't it?

It's not.

A *New York Times Magazine* profile on Ashlyn noted the scars on her hands from previous mishaps and described her parents' constant fear for her safety. When people who feel no pain fracture their bones or dislocate their joints, they may keep moving, worsening their injuries. Accumulating damage can lead to disability and surgery to amputate their limbs.[2]

We don't have to *like* pain. When it gets out of control—like from arthritis or chronic backache—we need to treat the cause. But we must acknowledge that we have it for a reason. Oddly enough, pain in reasonable amounts can improve our quality of life.

The same is true of your fear of death. If anxiety about dying keeps you from enjoying your life, it's a problem. But you shouldn't try to lock your awareness of death in a box or sweep every trace of it from your mind.

For starters, you may not be able to eradicate your fear of death any more than you can turn off your ability to feel pain.

In his book *Staring at the Sun: Overcoming the Terror of Death,* Stanford University professor emeritus and psychotherapist Irvin Yalom, MD, noted: "... We can never completely subdue death anxiety; it is always there, lurking in some hidden ravine of the mind."[3]

It's hardwired into us. You can take actions that are contrary to your fear of death—say, if you have to rescue a loved one from a burning building or jump your motorcycle over a row of buses for a TV special—but it's not reasonable to expect that you can completely ignore the presence of your mortality.

Secondly, respecting the dreadful power of your death provides benefits. When you live with the awareness that death will someday turn off the faucet that's supplying you with time, you're less likely to waste the stream that's flowing into your hands.

This notion came up during a chat I had one spring day with Victor Strecher, PhD, a University of Michigan professor who was driving across the countryside on a weekend road trip.[4]

When his daughter Julia was a baby, a virus damaged her heart, and she needed a transplanted heart to replace it. "Her very likely death when she was a baby started us to think, 'How could we help her live the biggest life possible?'" Dr. Strecher told me. Yet as he wrote in his book *Life on Purpose: How Living for What Matters Most Changes Everything,* "We'd also need to approach life with her in a whole new way—in a way that assumed she might die at any moment."

So they began creating a deliberate, purposeful life for themselves. "We're all on this planet for a brief period of time. Why are we sitting around watching what the Kardashian sisters are doing?" he asks.

Julia needed a second heart transplant at age 9. And when she was a 19-year-old nursing student, her heart stopped working again. Her life had reached its end. Over time, Dr. Strecher began taking his own life's purpose to a bigger stage. Along with his day job, which is researching ways to change people's health behaviors, he now tries to help *others* find their purpose in life.

The Immortal, a short story by Argentinian author Jorge Luis Borges, provided a source of inspiration for him.

The story's main character finds a magical river that grants immortality to all who drink from it. But he discovers that when you're immortal, you feel no motivation to get up and actually *use* your life. You don't help others with their challenges. You don't get anything done. It's a pretty miserable way to live. When the immortals in the story hear of a different river that will break this curse, they roust themselves up and go looking for it.[5]

If we deny that we're going to die, or we allow ourselves to overlook the death that will one day take away everything we have, the same thing happens, Dr. Strecher says. We lose an important source of motivation to live to the fullest. And when life nears its end, we may wish we'd used our limited supply differently.

"The fact that we're mortal beings gives great value to our lives. This is an idea in Buddhism, and it's true in life as well," says David Zuniga, PhD, a clinical psychologist at the MD Anderson Cancer Center in Houston. He brings several other perspectives that make for a lively conversation about death, as well. He's an ordained Zen Buddhist priest, and he worked for more than a decade as a hospice chaplain.[6]

"As Americans, we're all about quantity. But with life, it's really, really, really about *quality,* not just quantity," Dr. Zuniga says. "When you can embrace the fact that 'I am of the nature to die, my wife and children are of the nature to die, my parents and everyone I love is impermanent, and in 100 years, everyone I know will probably have died,' when you can sit with the totality of that, then everything in your existence becomes more important and more precious."

Embracing these truths doesn't mean you have to *like* them. Think of it more as *accepting* them. For you, that embrace begins today, as in right now. (Go ahead—give death a hug!) The time has come to:

- *Learn* how to carry an ongoing awareness of death that inspires you, rather than making you panic.

- *Break through* your denial that your time will someday end. People's unwillingness to acknowledge death can be "stunning," Dr. Zuniga says. "I was working with a patient who was emaciated with cancer and couldn't walk anymore. He said, 'Dave, I just don't think I'm going to die!'" But the man died the next day. "This person's denial is understandable. We live in a generally death-denying culture. It's a process to embrace our mortality," he says. But, "embracing death with insight and even some joy is possible."

- *Discover* a way to honor and respect death's role so you can learn from it. The end of life offers opportunities for growth and discovery . . . but not everyone finds them.

We naturally fear death to varying degrees, but we can also rise above it so we can still see it, but we don't feel overwhelmed by it.

Eight Ways to Adjust Your Outlook on Death

Starting a new relationship with your mortality isn't as easy as flipping a switch. But you can make a number of adjustments, both small and large, that will move you in the right direction.

In general, thinking about your death requires you to think about your life, since the two are tightly intertwined. To die happy, you must live well. But to live well, you must acknowledge and appreciate that death will happen to everyone, including you. The following activities will help you do that, redirecting you toward a more intentional and rewarding life.

Scan Yourself for Death Anxiety

If the thought of discussing your will with your spouse makes you agitated, or the idea of playing the lighthearted "death questions" game in Chapter 1 fills you with dread, you might have death anxiety.

For a small number of people, death anxiety hampers their daily lives. In 1969, 3.3 percent of people reported an "intense fear of death." More recently, nearly 4 percent told researchers they are "much more nervous" about death or dying than most people, and nearly 10 percent said they were "somewhat" more nervous.[7, 8]

Death anxiety becomes a problem when it provokes you to avoid situations that touch on illness or death, causes significant worry, or keeps you from enjoying your life, according to University of Manitoba, Canada, psychologists Patricia Furer, PhD, and John Walker, PhD. As mentioned in the previous chapter, excessive death anxiety often goes hand in hand with hypochondria and other types of anxiety, such as panic disorder.[9]

If you think death anxiety has become a problem for you, discuss your concerns with a mental health professional. The problem can be treatable with the following strategies, according to an overview that Drs. Furer and Walker wrote for the *Journal of Cognitive Psychotherapy.*

Reduce your excessive anxiety-related behaviors. People with health anxiety and death anxiety may frequently check on their physical well-being (like by examining moles or weighing themselves over and over); seek reassurance (perhaps by visiting the doctor or looking up symptoms online); or use "safety behaviors" (for example, by carefully following superstitions). A counselor or therapist may help you set goals that encourage you to rely on these behaviors less frequently.

Make yourself think about death. Contemplating death-related reminders may, over time, help you manage your anxiety about death. Try reading the obituaries in a newspaper, visiting a cemetery, or writing a short story envisioning the end of your life. Since doing your end-of-life planning is an important step toward reaching your version of a "good death," reducing your anxiety in this manner can also have practical benefits.

Trade in your excessive fear for something better. A little unease about death is okay. But when it's taking up too much space in your mind, try to turn your vision to something happier.

"When people are troubled by fear of death, their attention is often diverted from a focus on enjoying life," Drs. Furer and Walker write. Take time every day for activities that celebrate your life, rather than stewing over your demise. Chase your dog around the yard. Express yourself through art.

Savor a fine dinner. Feed your joy of living so it grows and flowers, and let your fear of death wither from lack of attention.

Think About Where You Were Before You Were Born

Here's a thought that might comfort you if you're nonreligious or you otherwise believe that once you die, you won't exist elsewhere in a different form. It dates back to Epicurus, a Greek philosopher who died around 270 BC. (Cause of death: kidney stones.)[10]

Start with this: According to NASA, the universe is roughly 13.8 billion years old. This is the length of time that transpired before you were born. Think back on this period before you existed. Do you remember it?[11]

Are you curious whether you were eager to be born, or whether you were bored while you marked the millennia in a sea of darkness? Do you feel like you missed some excitement on Earth a million years before you were born? No? Then why should you worry about what happens during the eternity that follows after your death?

"I have personally found it comforting on many occasions to think that the two states of nonbeing—the time before our birth and the time after death—are identical and that we have so much to fear about the second pool of darkness and so little concern about the first," Dr. Yalom writes in *Staring at the Sun*.

If you feel that your lifetime represents a period in which you step out of the night for just a second—like someone walking through the bright circle under a streetlight—then how are you going to use this time? Will you be lost in worry about returning to the darkness? Or will you see all you can during this illuminated moment?

Be Stoic About It

Stoicism is another school of thought, started in Greece around 300 BC, that still offers powerful strategies for coping with death in our modern age.[12]

Stoics looked at the natural world around them and saw that plants, animals, and humans alike "are born, they develop, mature and age, and then decrepitude sets in and death occurs," says William O. Stephens, PhD, professor of philosophy and classical studies at Creighton University in Omaha,

Nebraska. "This is part of a natural cycle that has been going on forever. It's always going to happen, and it's foolish not to recognize that."

Epictetus, a prominent Stoic, looked to food as a source of metaphor. The vine thickens and matures, then it sprouts grapes. When dried, those grapes become raisins. "If you desire for grapes never to turn into raisins, you desire for the universe to be different than it is," Dr. Stephens says. "To be human, among other things, is to be mortal. We were given birth by the universe, and our lives are on loan. If you desire to be immortal, what you're actually desiring is not to be a human being."

One more point about Stoicism, then we'll turn to the take-home message. Think about how long you've been reading this chapter. Maybe 10 minutes? How many people in the United States died during that time? Do you grieve the deaths of these strangers? Probably not. When an acquaintance's grandparent dies, are you sad? Perhaps a bit, at most.

(Oh, by the way, the answer is 50. That's how many Americans died in the past 10 minutes.)[13]

But when one of these deaths is your loved one, it hits you harder. "The Stoics say that's because you didn't remind yourself all along that your loved ones are aging and will die," Dr. Stephens says.

The solution is to continually remind yourself that everything around you is temporary, but with an attitude of *appreciation,* not fear. Start expressing gratitude for your houseplants, your pets, your loved ones, and your own life throughout the day, with the knowledge that they're all here for a short time, he says. How many parents buy their toddlers a goldfish because it's a guaranteed way to experience death in a tiny, educational dose . . . and how many of us forget this lesson?

Take a close look at the goldfish, and marvel at the sunlight flashing off its body. Savor the warmth of the coffee cup that someday may break in the sink. Enjoy your summer vacation. Be mindful of the joy inherent in being alive and sharing that life with your loved ones, he says.

"When you love mortal human beings and remember they're mortal—when you remind yourself of their vulnerability to illness, injury, even death—it allows you to realize that you must not take them for granted," he says.

So remind yourself to be awake and aware! Create a mantra that you'll regularly repeat to yourself—something along the lines of, "This is beautiful or precious to me, and I should appreciate it because it's temporary." Too many people around you don't.

Assume You'll Be Better Prepared

If you imagine your final moments, you're probably picturing yourself as you are right now, suddenly torn from your present surroundings and placed minutes away from death. Of course that's a frightening scenario—it's like an icy plunge into a scary future.

In real life, most of us will transition gradually from decent health to whatever end-of-life state awaits us, as you saw in those "death trajectories" on pages 3 and 4. The future version of yourself who will die will likely have time to prepare for what's happening.

This little realization emerged as I was speaking with Nicholas Carleton, PhD, associate professor of psychology at the University of Regina, Canada. We were discussing "intolerance of uncertainty" (in other words, the fear of the unknown), which is his professional focus.[14]

Then we veered off topic for a bit.

Dr. Carleton suspects that any part of you that heads off into Whatever Comes Next—like your soul—will also be better prepared to handle the situation than you currently are.

"One of two things has to be true: You pass away and some version of your consciousness goes to some version of heaven, hell, or limbo. If some part of you goes beyond death, *that* part of you will interact with that reality with whatever capacities it'll have, and there's probably no way to prepare yourself for what that will be like. In the same way that you learned how to cope with this reality, you'll learn how to cope with the next one," Dr. Carleton says.

"The other possibility is that your consciousness ceases. If you're aware that your consciousness is ceasing, the most terrifying components of that experience will only last for a few minutes, then there'll be nothing. In which case, there will be no *you* to try to grapple with the absence of you," he says. "If those are my only two options, then I'm okay with either of them."

Brush with Mortality Helped Woman Make Plan to Comfort Loved Ones

As Donna Belk lay on a hospital gurney in her midthirties, neither she nor her doctors realized she had an ectopic pregnancy. This condition—in which an embryo grows outside of the uterus—can be fatal in rare cases. For Belk, it nearly was.

"I was in a lot of pain, but then the pain started to slowly ebb away. As the pain lightened, I became more comfortable and felt very loved and warm," she says. "All of a sudden I was outside of my body. Then a tunnel started to form around me. The feelings of peacefulness and love continued to increase. Then the thought occurred to me, 'Ah, I know what's going on—I'm dying!'"

She felt a pang of fear. Belk was a single mother, and she worried what would happen to her two daughters if she died. That was her last memory until she woke up again.

Now when she thinks about death, it's with a sense of anticipation. "There's no fear of it. There's actually a longing for it, but not in a suicidal way." For her, the feeling is akin to looking forward to seeing a long-lost lover again.

Give Thought to All That You Will Leave Behind

Another source of comfort that Dr. Yalom espouses is the notion of *rippling.* That means making an impact on the world that keeps traveling after you're gone—like the ripples that still move outward long after a stone splashes and disappears into a pond.

There are plenty of ways that leave behind evidence that we existed, from making babies to donating money for a college to name a building after us. (Ultimately, both only exist temporarily, even the building.) But we also waste many opportunities to create ripples that require a lot less time than raising kids and cost a *lot* less than that donation.

The kind word or action you direct to a stranger at a low point could turn his life around. The backpack filled with school supplies you donate could provide an

Until that meeting arrives, the Austin, Texas, woman is living deliberately. When fears, grudges, or regrets arise in her mind, she examines them to see if she can resolve them now so they don't pop up on her deathbed. She bought a plot in a "green" cemetery, and she quizzes her daughters about her end-of-life wishes. ("So, if the doctors want to intubate me, what will you say?")

Belk has also made several mementos that she hopes will help her loved ones during their grieving process.

"I made a notebook that my family and friends can read if I have a lingering death and they're sitting vigil with me," she says. "I included poems and meditations that are significant to me, and in it I've written notes like 'If you're reading this, remember how much I love you' and 'If you have any regrets or felt you did something wrong, all I have for you is love.'"

She also made a shawl that might someday serve as a stand-in when she's gone. "I traced outlines of my arms and sewed them onto a big heart and quilted it," she says. "I made two of them for my daughters to wrap around themselves and feel me after I'm gone."

early toehold for a young innovator who will someday change the world. Or you could develop and share a terrific new idea . . . and ideas can never be destroyed.

Every day, ask yourself this question: "Are my ripples improving my surroundings or causing harm? Are the gifts I have—my creativity, smarts, morals, and ethics—reverberating out into the world, or am I keeping them to myself?"

This, too, is a Stoic perspective, Dr. Stephens says. The most important part of you isn't your *body,* a container that will break down and generate offensive smells. That container was made with an eventual expiration date.

"Worms and insects have bodies, too. Despite how impressed we are with our Olympic athletes, what's really special about humans is our capacity for reason and understanding," he says. Using our sense of reason, we can cultivate wisdom, justice, self-control, and generosity. "*That's* what is best about human beings, and those virtues can be passed on from our parents and teachers and mentors to us. As long as you retain those virtues inside you, your loved one lives on."

And if you pass on your most important values to others, so will you.

Changing Funeral Customs Allow You to Rejoin Nature

Some methods of managing your remains allow your body to spread out into the environment through plants and animals.

Cremation is rapidly becoming the most common method that people choose for the disposition of their bodies. In 2005, only 32 percent chose cremation. In 2017, that number has leaped to an estimated 52 percent, and by 2030, more than 70 percent of people may pick this option, according to the National Funeral Directors Association.[15]

If you opt for this route, your cremains could be placed into a stone bench in your garden or scattered on land or sea, depending on local laws. Or your powdery remains can be mixed into a structure that's dropped onto a coral reef to foster underwater life. For something completely different, they can also be compressed into a diamond.

If you want to be buried, you have several options aside from the customary approach, in which your embalmed body is sealed forever within a reinforced concrete vault. One of these options is the increasingly popular "green burial." With this approach, your body goes into a biodegradable container, which is then buried in a natural setting (think trees and tall grass). As nature completes its ancient process, your body becomes a source of sustenance for creatures that carry you out into the environment.

An Italian venture is taking this idea further. Currently, the Capsula Mundi project is developing egg-shaped "pods" to hold ashes or even your entire body. The idea is to lower the pod containing your remains into the ground, then plant a tree of your choosing atop it. Later, the tree could serve as a living memorial for your loved ones to gather around to celebrate your memory. In a sense, *you* would be there, too, alive in their presence.[16]

Think About a Promise behind the Pain

Newburyport, Massachusetts, was founded in 1764, so its cemeteries are really old, at least as far as American cemeteries go. While looking at a cluster of headstones in a graveyard there, hospice chaplain Kerry Egan, author of *On Living,* had a powerful realization.[17]

The stones marked the graves of a father, mother, and several children who had died in quick succession. "On one of the gravestones, I read something that I've never seen before or since. It basically said, 'We don't understand why you're doing this, God. Why are you doing this?' I felt like I could feel this woman's anguish screaming out hundreds of years later. It was still palpable," she told me.

"The New Testament says God is love. It's an equal sign: God = love. If you take that to be true, which I do, then there has to be something more. If God is love, this pain cannot be all there is. Because that's not the experience of love."

If you believe that a loving and benevolent creator made you for a reason, what is that reason? For what purpose would such a creator cause you to die and to face other suffering and losses before that time?

Furthermore, what's the bigger plan, and how will your painful life experiences and your death fit into it? Regardless of your religious belief—or whether you have one—this question is an important one to consider.

Distract Yourself with Something Better

For Chicago physician Alex Lickerman, MD, 2007 was a memorable year. In January, he needed surgery for appendicitis. The next day, he returned to the hospital in severe pain. He was bleeding internally after the procedure, and another surgery revealed that he'd lost half his blood volume.[18]

A few weeks later, he developed a blood clot in his lung, as well as a stubborn bacterial infection in his digestive system. Later, a mental health professional diagnosed him with PTSD brought on by his quick succession of health threats.

His brush with mortality left him shaken. Obviously, he knew that someday he would die, but now this abstract idea felt real. As he wrote in his book *The Undefeated Mind,* "Ultimately, being ill brought me to the realization, contrary to what I'd always believed in my heart, that there was nothing special about me at all. Like everyone else, I was only a piece of meat that would eventually spoil."[19]

Create a Ripple That Comforts Loved Ones and Strangers Alike

Want to confront your fear of death, kick-start an important conversation with your family, and maybe rescue enough people to fill 2½ school buses?

Make a public pledge to donate your organs and tissues after you die.

Organ transplants add length and richness to recipients' lives. In 2015, nearly 31,000 transplanted hearts, livers, lungs, kidneys, and other organs saved Americans from an early death, restored their function, or freed them from their attachment to dialysis machines.[20]

If you share your organs when you go, you can save up to eight people's lives. If you donate other tissues, like your corneas, heart valves, and bones, you can help restore function to a crowd of 100 more.[21]

By making this decision, you signal that you've taken an important step toward managing your fears about dying. One study, which compiled earlier research on the public's attitudes toward organ donation after death, found that "those who feared thinking or talking about death . . . were often reluctant to consider the issue of organ donation."[22]

Other research has found that organ donation doesn't just give a gift to strangers—it may provide comfort to the grieving loved ones you leave behind. "I think it gives me something more to think about besides death. This has diverted my thoughts to something positive," one family member of a donor said. "It gives some meaning to an otherwise meaningless tragedy," said another.[23]

Ready to pledge this meaningful gift? You can register in less than a minute at Organize.org. (You may find this quicker and more convenient than going to your Department of Motor Vehicles.) Then go tell your loved ones, since they'll have the final say on allowing the donation to happen.

A long-practicing Buddhist, he's been seeking ways to come to terms with his mortality, though it's a work in progress. "Today, the best answer I can come to is that I think the best way to deal with the fear of death is to *deny* it," he says. However, this isn't an unwise, harmful type of denial that keeps you from planning for your death, or the kind of denial that compels you to ignore a lump that could be treatable if you report it to your doctor early enough.

Instead, it's denying your fear a chance to grow by starving it of space. Want to keep weeds out of your lawn? Be sure the grass is so dense and healthy that they don't have room to take root. Similarly, "the best way to deny your fear of death is to live so vibrantly and excitedly that your thoughts are drawn away from death because you're so engaged in living a life that's interesting and fulfilling," Dr. Lickerman explains.

How do you live that vibrant, interesting, and fulfilling life? It all comes down to one simple word. And that word will be unveiled in italics in the next sentence.

Discover Why You're Here

For Dr. Lickerman, a central approach to living better in the face of death is to live a life of *meaning*. We'll explore how to create meaning in the next chapter. But first, let's introduce ourselves to this concept.

Michael MacKenzie and Roy Baumeister of Florida State University offered a nice overview in the 2014 book *Meaning in Positive and Existential Psychology*.[24] You can think of your life's meaning as the way you interpret how its different elements are put together. These elements include yourself, of course, as well as your job; your spouse, children, and other family members; your religious beliefs; and your hobbies and leisure activities.

Meaning helps you behave consistently and predictably over the long term. You're not lurching back and forth impulsively through your life. You have explanations for the things that are happening to you and guidance for your decisions and choices.

Your need for meaning goes hand in hand with your need for values, MacKenzie and Baumeister write. Your values help you decide whether an action feels right or wrong. You may derive your values from many places, including your religious beliefs or the laws of your country. If your actions consistently match your values, you're more likely to feel good about your choices. You're also less likely to feel guilty about things you've done when you come to the end of your life.

Your meaning gives you strength and resilience to manage the adversities that life puts in your path. Dr. Lickerman told me his meaning—or in his words, his mission—is to alleviate suffering wherever he sees it. Since he's a doctor, his job puts him in a great position to fulfill that mission. But his meaning influences other parts of his life, as well. He devotes some of his spare time to writing, which he hopes will guide people he'll never meet. As a parent, he wants to instill values in his son that encourage him to help other people, too.

After 21 years of practicing medicine, Dr. Lickerman has been present at many patients' final days. "I've heard a lot of people talk about how foolish they were to care about things that now seemed unimportant to them. They may also wonder whether they made a contribution to society," he says.

"If you get to the end of your life and feel like it wasn't meaningful, or that you wasted it, or that you didn't fulfill your potential, I can't imagine the suffering you'd have."

The Not-So-Predictable Link between Your Religion and Your Fear of Death

Religion can provide multiple layers of comfort in your life. You may look to it for guidance when you need to make decisions; reassurance that you have an eternal reward waiting for you after you die; or an opportunity to spend time with like-minded friends every week.

But what religion *doesn't* necessarily do is help you cope with a fear of death. Studies looking at the association between religious practice and attitudes toward death reveal conflicting findings.

For example, a questionnaire found that, among 130 worshippers at an Episcopalian church in New York, only the beliefs that God exists and an afterlife awaits were linked to less death anxiety and greater acceptance of dying. Other factors and practices, like more frequent prayer or church attendance, or looking to religion for guidance in daily decisions, didn't seem to reduce death fears.[25]

A study from Wellesley College in Massachusetts found that a combination of being strongly religious and having a strong belief in a pleasant afterlife may help reduce your fear of death. However, another finding was that people with lukewarm religious beliefs had the greatest fear of death, compared to people with either high or low religious beliefs. (Perhaps such people may worry more about punishment in the afterlife but feel they don't have a way to escape it, the authors note.)[26]

Another study—this one of college students in the United States, Malaysia, and Turkey—found that being more religious tends to be linked with a *greater* fear of death. The authors theorized that the beliefs emphasized in your religion can influence your death fears. Do you see God as forgiving or vindictive? Does your religion require you to follow a lot of rules or practice a lot of rituals, or do you have more leeway in how you honor your faith? Does attaining an eternal reward take a lifetime of effort, or can you achieve it late in life?[27]

In short, your spiritual beliefs and religious practices may relieve or increase your death anxiety. In Chapter 4, we'll return to this topic to discuss how you can get the greatest sense of meaning from your religious practice.

LIVE WELL, DIE HAPPY EXERCISES
Chapter 2

How much fear does death hold for you right now? Did you find any tools that might address any death anxiety you've been harboring? I'd like to direct your thoughts to the following activities that may help you make more progress.

Please bookmark this page, and take note of the factors that you rate a 6 or higher below. Interspersed throughout the book, you'll find solutions for all of these death-related fears that might help ease your concerns.

1. On a scale of 1 (very little) to 10 (a lot), estimate how much distress you feel about the following ideas related to dying.

I may feel pain or discomfort during my final days.

1	2	3	4	5	6	7	8	9	10

I'll be forgotten after I'm gone.

1	2	3	4	5	6	7	8	9	10

I'll die without accomplishing my goals.

1	2	3	4	5	6	7	8	9	10

My family will suffer financially without me.

1	2	3	4	5	6	7	8	9	10

I have old disagreements I haven't resolved or damaged relationships I haven't repaired.

1	2	3	4	5	6	7	8	9	10

My loved ones won't cope well with my death.

1	2	3	4	5	6	7	8	9	10

I'll die feeling that I wasted my life.

1	2	3	4	5	6	7	8	9	10

No one will be around to take care of me at the end.

1	2	3	4	5	6	7	8	9	10

2. Do any of your family members or close friends display a sense of meaning or purpose in their daily lives? If so, talk to them about how they came upon it; how they apply it in their work, personal, or family activities; and what benefits they get from it. _____

_____

_____

_____

_____

_____

3. If you can safely donate blood, consider giving a pint. How does the thought of a stranger walking around with your donated blood make you feel? What else could you do today—large or small—to feel connected to fellow humans in a meaningful way? _____

_____

_____

_____

_____

_____

4. How well do your religious beliefs, or your secular outlook, as may be the case, protect you from excessive worry about death? If dying distresses you, make an appointment with your pastor or worship leader to see if your religion offers a source of comfort you've overlooked. Or go online to see how prominent atheist or humanist thinkers—there's a growing number of them—cope with thoughts of death. _____

_____

_____

_____

_____

_____

CHAPTER 3

Pursue a Life
of Meaning

The overcrowded train carrying prisoner number 119,104 slowed in the pre-dawn light as it reached its destination. "Auschwitz!" one of his fellow passengers cried out in alarm. Gradually, the industrial-scale horror of the camp revealed itself as the train crawled forward.

As he was processed into the camp, the prisoner, a psychiatrist approaching middle age, was quickly separated from his most prized possession: an unpublished manuscript containing his ideas about psychotherapy.

Over the next few years, as he was shuttled between work camps, the prisoner's pregnant wife and parents died. He dug ditches in the frozen ground, clothed only in rags to cover his skeletal frame, his feet sometimes so swollen he could barely walk. His companions fell steadily away. Death could come for the most trivial of reasons: an official pointing his finger toward the crematorium, a too-long trek to the work site, or an outbreak of contagion.

But he endured until April 1945. When the camp was liberated, among the survivors who emerged was prisoner 119,104. His name was Viktor Frankl.

He developed great insight into the core drive that keeps humanity going, even when life is unimaginably awful. Throughout his suffering, Frankl made observations and took notes on hidden scraps of paper.

Once freed, he poured out his thoughts during a 9-day writing frenzy. The resulting book would sell more than 10 million copies during the next 50 years of his life. Its title: *Man's Search for Meaning.*[1,2]

According to Frankl, we must have meaning. If we lack it, we'll look for it. If we're without it for too long, we suffer. "There is much wisdom in the words of Nietzsche: 'He who has a *why* to live for can bear almost any *how,*'" Frankl wrote. "In the Nazi concentration camps, one could have witnessed that those who knew that there was a task waiting for them to fulfill were most apt to survive."

Today's research continues to confirm that having a sense of meaning is linked to better physical health, well-being, and even longevity.

- Researchers who compiled the results of earlier studies in 2016 found that among 136,000 people, those with a higher sense of purpose were 17 percent less likely to have a cardiovascular event like a heart attack or stroke.[3]

- According to Belgian researchers who surveyed people with chronic illnesses like arthritis or low back or neck pain, those who felt their lives had more meaning also reported greater well-being. In this study, "meaning" was a measure of how significant and purposeful their lives felt.[4]

- Another study asked more than 6,100 adults, ages 20 to 75, three questions that measured the purposefulness of their lives: Do I wander aimlessly through life? Do I just live for the current day? Have I done everything there is to do in life? During 14 years of follow-up, those with a higher sense of purpose were about 15 percent less likely to die. It didn't matter if they were young, middle-aged, or old, or employed or retired—greater purpose was linked to a longer life.[5]

Let's pause for a minute. Are you zoning out at the mention of "meaning"? Are your eyes glazing over with talk about your "purpose"? If so, it's completely understandable. Yes, "meaning in life" can become a deep concept. It may seem like the domain where mystics and New Agey folks gather. You've probably seen *way* too many dumb newspaper comics about it, invariably featuring a guru atop a mountain.

Finding your life's meaning doesn't have to look like any of these images. Defining your version of meaning can be simple and straightforward. *Living* a life of meaning doesn't have to be complicated, either. Once you've developed your sense of meaning, you'll have a handy tool—a compass, of sorts—to guide you through a more satisfying life, whether you're in a comfortable and prosperous phase or you're suffering through the loss and distress that all humans will face.

Follow these eight steps for zeroing in on your meaning, and you'll start wringing more value from your time on Earth.

Step 1: Learn What Life Meaning Is

"Life is short. It's easy to waste and hard to use," said Michael Steger, PhD, associate professor of psychology at Colorado State University, during a TEDx talk that made the rounds online. Since that statement is a pretty good way to sum up this entire book, I chatted with him via Skype to discuss solutions to it. He made a witty and compelling case for why we need to create a sense of direction in our lives.[6]

Dr. Steger is well-known in the field of meaning, which he describes as containing three components.

You have a purpose—or several purposes. Some people think of meaning and purpose as the same thing, but Dr. Steger sees purpose as a path to meaning. "I usually define purpose as a set of large, overarching, open-ended things we're striving for in life: 'I want to be a good parent; I want to make the world a better place; I want to fully explore my potential; I want to make a difference.' It's the journey, not the outcome, that matters when it comes to purpose." In other words, even if Bill and Melinda Gates die before their foundation's goal of eradicating malaria is complete, they'll probably feel that their time and effort were well spent.

Victor Strecher, PhD—whom you met in the previous chapter—told me he has four domains, or areas, of purpose.

"I have a *personal* purpose, a *family* purpose, a *work* purpose, and a *community or global* purpose. Put together, my entire purpose is to enjoy love and beauty; to be an engaged husband, father, and grandfather; to teach every one of my students as if they're my own child; and to be an engaged leader and to reach people to help them find greater purpose in life."

Your life makes sense. When your purpose is well defined, the meaning that grows from it gives you the feeling that "I have a big picture of my life that includes me and the rest of the world. If you don't have that, then life is unpredictable, and things don't ever work out like you think they will. You feel alienated and outside of everything," Dr. Steger says.[7]

Your meaning also helps you feel that your life is unfolding like a coherent story. The plot makes sense, actions lead to foreseeable outcomes, and the characters around you act in ways that you can generally anticipate. (Have you ever seen a movie series where the sequels don't make sense when you watch them in order? A meaningful life is the opposite of that.)

You recognize that your life is worth it. "For the nerds among us who are trying to figure out this topic, those first two components alone don't seem like they're enough. I've settled on 'life is significant' as the third," Dr. Steger says. "Imagine you're on your deathbed. Someone asks the question, 'Was it worth it?' Yeah, it's significant, it's worthwhile, my life has some sort of value. It doesn't have anything to do with *why* it's worthwhile or *how* you managed to create value."

Your life's meaning is an ongoing presence that steers you through the everyday hassles and the big highs and lows. It permeates the different areas of your life. It's steady, yet it can evolve over time. It's a crucial element of your story.

The great part about your life's meaning is that *you* get to decide it. There is no right or wrong answer, as long as it's significant for you. The flip side of that, however, is that *only* you get to decide it. No one else can do it for you.

Step 2: Learn What Life Meaning Isn't

The reason we're here, according to esteemed thinker Tenzin Gyatso, is "to be happy." (Haven't heard of him? He's better known as the Dalai Lama.)[8] But please note that meaning and happiness are two different ambitions that can work at cross-purposes with each other.

A 2013 study from the *Journal of Positive Psychology* explored the differences between a meaningful life and a happy life, based on a series of surveys that asked participants to rate their meaning and happiness.[9]

The two often went hand in hand. However, the researchers painted a picture of how it's possible to have a very meaningful life that's not so happy. It might look like this: You "sacrifice (your) personal pleasures in order to participate constructively in society," they wrote. Or maybe you spend a lot of time thinking about your past challenges and imagining the future, or you're more of a giver than a taker. Frankl found meaning in the concentration camps, but happiness was scarce.

On the other hand, you can have a happier life that's not so meaningful. Perhaps your life is "relatively shallow, self-absorbed, or even selfish." Maybe you avoid challenging yourself very hard.

"Meaning and happiness seem to follow different patterns. What feeds into meaning are a lot of things about connection and what it all adds up to," Dr. Steger says. But factors like "Do I get the things I want today? Are people giving me too much crap?" can affect your happiness. "If people don't give me crap today, that doesn't make life feel more meaningful, but it'll be a better day for me," he says.

If you had to choose just one to support a life that flourishes over time, he says, then "meaning is a better driver of that than happiness is. Because life is messy and we don't get everything we want, it's good to have meaning to get value out of life when it's tough."

But you don't have to choose *either* meaning or happiness. You should have both, ideally adjusted to an optimal balance. You might look at meaning as eating a diet of fresh fruits and vegetables, whole grains, and lean meat to protect your overall health and improve your chances of a long life. Happiness, however, can be the thing that tastes good *now*—the box of candy at the movies, the scoop of ice cream, or the chicken that's breaded instead of grilled.

Note that happiness can grow from fast-acting pleasures, but it comes in other flavors, too. In his book *Life on Purpose,* Dr. Strecher explores the differences between two types of happiness. The ancient Greek philosophers called one *eudaimonia.* This is the happiness that comes from growth and self-exploration. It's more like a long-term contentment.[10]

The other, *hedonia,* is related to the word *hedonism:* It's the short-term pleasure that we might derive from eating, drinking, sex, and various vices. If when you wake up you groan as you remember the previous night's party, you were probably indulging in hedonia. This is the type of happiness that often drives behavior. In the modern world, "we've reduced our definition of happiness to the dopamine-driven experiences of pleasure. Eudaimonia sounds like a bit more work," Dr. Strecher writes.

To achieve stability, make the effort to ensure that your happiness and meaning work together. "A great life will have meaning and happiness in harmony so that both are happening at the same time, and you're not swinging back and forth. You're doing good things with your life, but you're also having fun," Dr. Steger says.

But as you're seeking the right balance of meaning and happiness, also seek out the ideal mix of these subtypes of happiness. In his book, Dr. Strecher pointed out a small study that found that these types of happiness may have very different effects in the body. The researchers asked 80 people about their sense of hedonic and eudaimonic well-being. People who were happier in a hedonic sense tended to be inclined to have greater inflammation in their bodies. This could raise one's risk of heart disease, cancer, and viral infections.[11]

As with diet and the food we eat, a well-balanced life of meaning and happiness may be key for our physical and mental health!

Step 3: Be Ready to Do More Searching Than Your Grandparents Did

A number of large surveys, both in the United States and abroad, suggest that the majority of us feel that our lives are meaningful. Across 132 countries, whether wealthy or developing, 91 percent of people said "yes" when pollsters asked them, "Do you feel that your life has an important purpose or meaning?"[12]

It's one thing to check "Yes, my life has meaning" on a form that someone hands you, but it's a different challenge to *define* your meaning or continue to find nourishment from it when your life gets hard. Perhaps now, especially.

Over the past century, we've seen big shifts in the social structures that historically provided meaning to the masses. Organized religion has fewer followers. Women are waiting longer to have kids, and parents are having fewer of them, compared to historical trends.[13, 14] You're less likely to spend decades working for one company. What it means to identify with either of our major political parties is changing.

Back when these institutions were more pervasive in everyday life and people conformed to them in similar patterns, you could look at the people next to you to see where they were deriving meaning, and then do the same as them, Dr. Steger says.

"I think of a lot of these big-system things as like the buffet for meaning. It's laid out there for you," he says. Discovering your meaning requires more work, though, "if suddenly things at the buffet start disappearing—if work disappears, if religion disappears, if social clubs disappear, if neighborhood disappears, if knowing everyone when you go shopping disappears from the buffet."

Step 4: Pick a Way the World Could Be Better

One way to begin cultivating your sense of meaning is to think about particular values you'd like to amplify in the world, and then live your life in a way that demonstrates these values. Some options to consider, according to Dr. Strecher, are community, kindness, relationships, vitality, or tradition.

You could also strive to bring more justice or love into the world. Or you could help alleviate hunger, or pollution, or even poor manners.

Is it possible to develop a sense of meaning that's purely about *your* comfort and enrichment? Can your meaning come from accumulating more money and power, or from building the nicest house on your block? Well, sure. It happens.

"Most people do not claim they derive meaning from selfish, materialistic, or petty things, but some do. It's not impossible," Dr. Steger says. Still, socially beneficial values "are the norm, not the exception. If we take a look at what philosophers say, the best kind of meaning is self-transcendent meaning. The data support that also, which is nice." (Self-transcendent is a way of saying that your meaning extends beyond yourself and to other people.)

Step 5: Assess Your Strengths

Next ask yourself this, "What is in my toolbox to help me act on those values?" Dr. Steger says, "Your strengths are the tools you're going to deploy to enact your values. In a sense, values (what you want to do) plus strengths (how you think you're going to do it) equals a sense of direction, purpose, and mission."

Are you intelligent in a way that solves problems? Do people often come to you seeking advice and counsel for their personal challenges? Are you good at connecting people to help fuse *their* strengths? Are you empathetic and caring? These may be strengths to tap into to support your values, which in turn will help sustain your life's meaning.

"Now, what's that look like over a 10-year span? What open-ended quest does that raise for you?" Dr. Steger asks.

Step 6: Write a Mission Statement, and Find Strategies to Support It

So far, you've determined the values that are important to you.

Then you looked within yourself for the strengths that will help you send those values out into the world.

The next step is to write a mission statement that incorporates your values and strengths.

Very often, businesses commonly have mission statements that drive their activities.

- **Google:** "... to organize the world's information and make it universally accessible and useful." Notice that the company's mission is *not* to provide a fast search engine. It long ago diversified to bring maps, medical research, and many other types of data to the globe's well-connected inhabitants.[15]

- **Tesla:** "... to accelerate the world's transition to sustainable energy." Previously, its mission statement referred to electric vehicles, but it has broadened its focus.[16, 17]

- **Mayo Clinic:** "To inspire hope, and contribute to health and well-being by providing the best care to every patient through integrated clinical practice, education, and research." Note that the world-renowned hospital seeks to improve patient care in part by educating its healthcare providers and conducting research. Its mission goes beyond just doing surgery and prescribing medications.[18]

- **Goodwill:** "... To enhance the dignity and quality of life of individuals and families by strengthening communities, eliminating barriers to opportunity, and helping people in need reach their full potential through learning and the power of work." If you thought Goodwill was there just to sell hand-me-down household items at steep discounts, you overlooked the organization's true mission.[19]

Note that each of these multimillion (or *billion*)-dollar companies is succeeding with a one-sentence mission statement of 8 to 35 words. You have a mission inside you. What sentence will summarize it?

You'll then need to identify strategies that support your mission.

In his book *The Undefeated Mind,* physician Alex Lickerman, MD, shares the story of a patient who was stricken with anxiety after being laid off from his job. Dr. Lickerman decided to help the patient discover his meaning (or in other words, his *mission*). "Once we figure out our mission, then we can turn value-creating activities that interest us into *strategies* with which we can accomplish it," Dr. Lickerman told him.[20]

A strategy is the action you take to support your mission. Strategies can and will fail, Dr. Lickerman says, so you'll need to be ready to adopt others as necessary.

You can lose your job. A project can fall apart. Friends and loved ones move away. You don't make the Olympic team. Thus, your strategy becomes impossible. But if you have an ongoing mission (or meaning) that stirs your heart, you'll bounce back with a new strategy that matches your changing abilities or resources.

If a sculptor's mission is "to fill the world with beauty," Dr. Lickerman writes, she can fulfill this mission even if her art doesn't sell or she becomes physically unable to shape the clay, since she can create beauty in other ways.

Step 7: Look to Others for Guidance

The practice of Buddhism requires devoting yourself to three important ideals, called The Three Jewels, says David Zuniga, PhD, a Texas psychologist who focuses on end-of-life issues. The first is the Buddha, or teacher. The second is the dharma, or the Buddha's teachings. The third is the Sangha, or your fellow practitioners.[21]

You can apply this "three jewel" concept to your life's pursuit of meaning even if you aren't Buddhist.

First, seek out people who can serve as teachers. Perhaps one could be a wise elder you admire in your community, someone who has led a meaning-driven life. Maybe it's your spiritual leader, a philanthropist in your city, or a single mother who has persevered through hard times. Or maybe a teacher is someone who has nurtured the life ingredients you find especially meaningful, like career, family, or personal development. Spend time with your teachers. Ask them questions. Learn from them.

Second, give thought to how the Buddhist values of kindness, compassion, generosity, and patient acceptance might support your life's meaning. These are good qualities for all of us to cultivate, regardless of what religion we may follow. (Or *not* follow: "Even atheists can be spiritual, and atheists can make great Buddhists," Dr. Zuniga says.)

Third, be active in a community of like-minded people who share your sense of purpose, Dr. Zuniga recommends. For example, if you were training for a marathon, you might join a running club so you'd have extra motivation to show up for a run because people you respect would be waiting for you. You would also have companionship and support over the long miles.

The same holds true as you pursue your sense of meaning. Seeing others deriving benefits from similar choices can reinforce your dedication to the path you've chosen.

There are other advantages to belonging to a like-minded community; remember from Chapter 1 that this sort of group membership also helps you reduce your fear of death.

Step 8: Stick with It

Once you've decided on your meaning/mission, make a vow to follow it, Dr. Lickerman recommends. Wishful thinking isn't enough, as it doesn't hold you directly responsible for making your pursuit of meaning happen.

"Making a vow, or determination, on the other hand, produces the opposite effect: It prevents us from expecting others to act on our behalf and from making excuses for our own inaction," he writes. So don't just write down your mission statement. *Commit* to it. Share it with the people close to you, and tell them about the strategies you'll deploy in pursuit of it.

There are certain challenges that no one else—your spouse, your boss, your parents, your teachers—will be able to solve. It will be up to you. Ultimately, you'll have the final say over whether you come to terms with the losses you face during your life. You will determine whether you forgive others or ask for forgiveness. Your experience at the end of life will be unique to you, as well. And so goes your search for meaning: Others may be able to assist, but you own the process of finding it and living it.

In the branch of Buddhism that Dr. Lickerman practices, encountering obstacles is "considered, paradoxically, the path to a life of 'comfort and ease.' For only in facing a strong enemy are we able to become strong ourselves," he writes. " . . . All of us have the capacity to make use of any circumstance, no matter how awful, to create value."

When you have a meaning—or purpose, or mission, as you choose to call it—you have a powerful tool that will help you live a vibrant and productive life until death ends it. Your life's meaning will also help you make sense of the painful moments you encounter, both while they're happening and in the future, when you review your life's story and think about what it all meant.

In the next section, you'll learn how to get the most meaning and happiness from eight possible uses of your time. You'll also discover how to make important adjustments to your habits and your attitudes that will boost your physical and emotional well-being over the coming years and decades.

To Find Meaning, Click Here

Need help finding your life's meaning? Try looking through your smartphone. Sometimes when Michael Steger, PhD, associate professor of psychology at Colorado State University, is teaching a workshop, he'll take the participants on a "meaning safari" in which he asks them to "take four pictures that capture your sense of what's meaningful about your life and world."

During his TEDx talk, Dr. Steger shared several photos that people found meaningful: a nature scene that encouraged a woman to stop and appreciate the moment. A tractor that reminded a young man of his family's farming heritage. A young man emptying a trash can ("This is my work . . . (as) a custodian. This is the first job that will not get me in trouble," he said).

Keep your camera ready today, and take a snapshot when you see something that represents your meaning, purpose, or mission, or even one of your values or strengths. Then share it with someone close to you, he urges. Describing to others why it's important will help you better understand it for yourself.

Plus, as you'll see later in this book, when you and your loved ones know the values that propel each of you and the qualities that give your lives meaning, you will all be in a much better position to make decisions that could determine whether or not you have a "good" death.

LIVE WELL, DIE HAPPY EXERCISES
Chapter 3

1. Off the top of your head, list the organizations and practices that provide your life with meaning—like religion, family, career, and hobbies. _____

_____

_____

_____

_____

_____

_____

2. List three people (either individuals you know or public figures) who seem to be using their lives for a particular purpose. _____

_____

_____

_____

_____

_____

_____

_____

3. Write some of the values you'd like to see amplified in the world. _____

_____

_____

_____

_____

_____

_____

4. Write some of the strengths you could use to broadcast these values into the world. _____

_____

_____

_____

_____

_____

_____

5. Write a mission statement to guide your life, incorporating your values and strengths. _____

_____

_____

_____

_____

_____

_____

6. List some *strategies* you could use to carry out your life's mission. In other words, what are specific actions you might take to follow your mission in different ways? _____

_____

_____

_____

_____

_____

_____

_____

Part 2

ADJUST YOUR PERSONAL SETTINGS

When you want to adjust your television, computer, smartphone, or any other complicated electronic device, you probably know where to go. Each of these gadgets has a control panel or settings page where you can make multiple modifications for your changing surroundings or needs.

Your life also needs regular calibrations to ensure that its different parts are working well together and providing the most meaning and happiness. But how often do you deliberately adjust it?

How often do you examine the question, "Do I need *more* of this activity or *less* of that one?" or "Do I see my surroundings clearly, or do I need to turn the dial on my focus?" or "Which of my health-related habits need fine-tuning?"

Now is a good time to ask these questions and make the appropriate adjustments. One way to make them more easily is to borrow from your electronic devices and create Personal Settings. You can come back to it periodically to retune your life. In this section, you'll learn how to adjust three core groups of settings so your life continually operates at peak performance.

1. **Your sources of meaning and happiness.** In Chapter 4, you'll adjust the time and energy you direct to eight important areas in your life.

2. **Your mind-set about the past, present, and future.** Four crucial adjustments discussed in Chapter 5 will help you feel more content with where you've *been,* where you *are,* and where you're *going.*

3. **Your health.** In Chapter 6, you'll learn to adjust your approach to your physical and mental well-being to help you live well in the face of age-related changes and chronic health conditions that often arise later in life.

CHAPTER 4

Adjust Your Time to Fit Your Life's Meaning

When you reach the end of your life, you may tell yourself, "Wow, that went fast!" But you know what's going to go *really* fast? The coming week. You'll have just 119 waking hours to get everything done in the next 7 days, and that's if you get by with 7 hours of sleep per night.

Some activities will be nonnegotiable: perhaps working to pay the bills, or caring for your family. Some things will feel good in the moment: eating a delicious meal, going on vacation, or having sex. Sometimes you'll just want to shut off your brain and forget your problems for as long as it takes to watch a couple of TV episodes, take a trip to the mall, or play a round of golf.

If you do it right, you can allocate your time each week so you're covering your daily demands, yet supporting your life's meaning and happiness. Then, when you look back someday, you're more likely to feel that you made good use of your life. It all came together to form a marvelous creation.

On the other hand, it's very easy for a sizable portion of those 119 hours to leak away in drips or evaporate like vapor each week. You don't use them to buy something lasting. They don't accumulate into anything bigger. They're just *gone*.

To live well and die happy, you'll need to devote *a significant portion of your time and attention* each week to meaningful uses.

The optimal way to spend *this* week is going to be very different from how you'll spend a week 10 years from now, or 10 years after that. That's because the people in your daily life are going to change. Your hobbies will change. You'll likely have a different job, or you'll be retired. Maybe you'll discover a passion for CrossFit or long-distance running, or maybe the opposite will happen—perhaps a knee injury or a chronic illness will limit your mobility.

So, your expenditure of time and focus will need to keep up with life's changes. If your main activity is caring for an ailing loved one, what will you do with your time when this person is gone? If a day-long bike ride is the only way you want to spend your Saturday, how will you respond if you develop a back problem that reduces the fun of riding?

You'll also need to *watch for unforeseen consequences* of how you're using your time. If your desire to provide for your family keeps you away from them until 8:00 p.m. every night, you're missing chances to create memories that build your legacy. Or you could give so much of yourself to volunteer work that you burn out. Or the activities you do for fun could actually be a way you're distracting yourself from serious problems.

You can categorize your 119 weekly hours into eight types of activities that may provide meaning and happiness.

1. Work
2. Close relationships, like with your spouse, family, and close friends
3. Spirituality/religion
4. Service to others
5. Self-improvement
6. Physical pleasures
7. Entertainment and travel
8. Acquiring money and possessions

At the end of this chapter, you'll find exercises that help you to fine-tune each of these areas. You can photocopy pages 79 to 83 or scan and print them, then adjust your activities and goals periodically.

Let's go through these eight uses of your weekly hours to discover how to get the most benefit from them today, and how to fit them into your meaningful life as it evolves.

Work: Charge Your Battery with a Powerful Calling

These days, we often refer to a career "calling" to mean that we have a passion for our work, says Bryan Dik, PhD, associate professor of counseling psychology at Colorado State University. If you feel passionate about your job, congratulations. Too few people do. But a calling means much more, and when your work meets the expanded definition of this concept, it will fit better into your life's meaning.[1]

A calling has three elements, Dr. Dik says. First, "it conveys there's a caller. For people of faith, that caller usually is God. But the concept can refer to any sources beyond the self—like your family or your legacy. You feel like, 'I'm set apart. I'm marked to do this work by something I can't even fully explain, but that is bigger than just me,'" Dr. Dik says.

Second, the purpose of your work aligns with your life's bigger story. "What I do all day is not separate from what matters most to me. It provides an opportunity for me to express a broader set of purpose," says Dr. Dik, coauthor of *Make Your Job a Calling*. Third, you feel that your work helps other people: "I do it not just because it makes me the happiest, but because I want to use my gifts to have a meaningful impact on the world around me."

Whether you're hunting for work or feeling content with your current 9-to-5, here's how to get the most meaning and happiness from your job.

Look within yourself. In his book, Dr. Dik shares the story of a police officer who heard the voice of God clearly tell him to leave his job to become a pastor. Though it took a lot of work to make the switch, he did well in his new career. [2]

This type of direct divine intervention doesn't figure into most people's career paths, Dr. Dik stresses. You can play a more active role in pursuing your calling by examining your strengths (like you did while looking for your life's meaning in the previous chapter).

"That includes your abilities, interests, values, and personality characteristics. When I talk to people who ask, 'How can I figure out my calling?' I tell them to look at how they're unique. How well is this job going to fit with how you're unique? Will this job allow you to swim with the current instead of against it?"

Also ask yourself what sorts of activities bring you joy. If you could spend your day doing anything, what would you do? Now dig deeper: What makes those activities appeal to you? As you look for work, seek a job that uses your strengths and provides these kinds of opportunities.

Ask questions. If you're in the market for a new job, the hiring manager will ask you questions at the interview. Be sure to do the same. Find out as much about the job and the workplace as you can. Ask the manager what your typical day will look like. What types of decisions will you make? Whom will you be interacting with? What skills and personality characteristics make someone good at this job? How will your contribution help the company?

And finally, ask *yourself* this big question: Can you clearly connect this job to your life's meaning or purpose? If the job is like a gearwheel that fits into the mechanism of a watch, it's a good candidate for your calling.

Look for meaning in your present job. If you're currently in a job you intend to keep, see if you can make some adjustments so it fits better into your big picture.

Some jobs are likely to simply feel inherently more meaningful than others, Dr. Dik says. These tend to give you freedom to make decisions; they require you to handle multiple tasks that use a variety of your skills; and they allow you to see the people you're helping. You might put medicine, nursing, or teaching in this category.

But it's possible to find meaning in jobs that don't necessarily appear to meet these criteria. Dr. Dik suggests an exercise called job crafting to help you make your current job more meaningful. First, list the tasks you perform each day under three headings, grouping them by whether they take a small, medium, or large amount of your time and attention. Now reorganize them to create a picture of what you'd *like* your job to become. Shift the tasks you most enjoy into the "large" category. Ideally, you'd like to do these tasks more often. If any of them seem to touch on the same theme, group them together and note how they're related.

Second, jot down a list of your values (the elements you need a job to provide in order for you to be satisfied); your interests (the things you do in the job that you enjoy); and your personality traits (specifically, the traits that most strongly define who you are). Then look at the themes that emerge from the group of tasks you'd like to do more often. Do any of these types of tasks connect to your values, interests, and personality? If so, *those* are the parts of your job that likely help make it a calling, Dr. Dik says.

Ask your boss if you can revise your job description to put more of your focus on these tasks. Perhaps you can trade some duties with a coworker. In the meantime, when you think about your job or describe it to others, focus on *these* parts of it.

Avoid the dark side. "I think it's more likely that people who approach work as a calling or who find all kinds of meaning in it end up struggling with work-life balance," Dr. Dik says. Workaholism can be a "dark side" of having a calling.

"If you feel so passionate about what you do for your job, and you feel like it's making an important impact on the world, it becomes easy to rationalize overinvesting in it. Sometimes people lose sight of the broader scope of what's important in life," he says.

To keep your work and personal life in balance, regularly set goals for what you want to accomplish in the other areas, or domains, that are important to you. Remind yourself that "this is the kind of family life I want to have. What do I need to do to ensure that I'm having that kind of marriage and that kind of relationship with my children? Start proactively pursuing those kinds of goals, and you can't help but make different choices about your work so you have time and energy for the other domains in your life," he says.

This, by the way, is the essence of this section of the Personal Settings exercises in this chapter: prioritizing what you want from each of the eight uses of your weekly hours, then allocating your time and attention accordingly.

Know when to make sacrifices and when to stop. During some periods in your life, investing more time in work may benefit your overall life plan, even if it intrudes into the other domains for a while. But return to the Personal Settings exercises as you meet career goals and ask yourself: "Is it now time to reinvest more of myself in some other area?"

In Dr. Dik's case, he had to sacrifice some family time to become a tenured professor. But the new job title brought him greater long-term job security and more freedom to seek meaning in his work. However, not everyone recognizes when enough is enough, career-wise.

Brush with Cancer Shifts Woman's Perspective on Work, Family, Community

After she got engaged at age 25, Melissa Keller had little time to celebrate with her fiancé.

A week later, the St. Louis woman was diagnosed with ovarian cancer. The couple's conversations turned from *when* they'd have kids to *how* they were going to have them.

"I went from the highlight of my life to my worst point," she says. Despite the fearsome reputation of ovarian cancer, her doctors thought her chances of survival were good. But she needed a hysterectomy, and she opted for 6 months of chemotherapy for added protection.

Though Keller was making good money at a Web site development company, she shifted course. "I thought, 'What kind of legacy will I leave? Am I cut out to just sit at a cubicle and have money, or is my priority something that's truly going to make a difference?'"

She returned to school and became a teacher. She began creating deeper, more meaningful connections with the people around her. Gardening helped her explore a newfound appreciation for the

"You can become addicted to achievement. Believe me, I've had colleagues who, no matter what accomplishment they're able to achieve, they can't look at it without thinking of others they haven't achieved yet. They organize their lives to achieve those accomplishments, and at the end of the day, it starts to ring hollow," he says, adding with a chuckle, "If you think about how you'll evaluate things on your deathbed, you may make some choices differently."

Regret over spending too much time at work often appears when people are on their deathbeds. Adjust your settings now so you won't rue your time management later.

---

environment, and it allowed her to nurture life in the vegetables, flowers, and trees she planted.

"The perspective you get on life after facing cancer is a gift. I think you feel things much more deeply than the average person. You have a much more emotional connection with everything in your life. You're driven by a sense of, 'Why wait to pursue your dreams?'" she says.

Time saw her fears of a cancer recurrence subside, though she grieved not being able to have children, especially around Mother's Day. Eventually, the couple adopted a newborn baby girl, Ruby. A few years later, they amicably parted ways.

Today, Keller stays busy teaching and co-parenting her 4-year-old. But she takes time to focus on the fleeting moments of goodness that catch her attention.

"If I see a beautiful sunset, I'll stop the car to enjoy it. A lot of people are yelling at their spouses; they're upset and not paying attention to their kids; and they're letting moments go by," she says. "It equates in my mind to using stuff and throwing it away without thinking about it. People can sort of throw away their lives without knowing it."

Tend to Your Spouse, Kids, and Other Close Relationships

In 2015, roughly 430,000 boys played high school soccer in the United States. Each of these players had a 5.7 percent chance of going on to play at an NCAA college. Out of this group, each had just a 1.4 percent chance of going on to Major League Soccer.[3]

Odds are similarly slim that your athletic teen will ever suit up as a professional football, baseball, basketball, or hockey player. It's likely that you're not really driving your kid to practices with a major-league career on your mind. But as you're planning your family's time, it's wise to ask yourself what your schedule *is* preparing your child to become, says Alexandra H. Solomon, PhD, clinical psychologist at The Family Institute at Northwestern University in Northbrook, Illinois.[4]

"We are parenting in a time of hyperintense focus on kids. I grew up in the 1970s and 80s, and our weekend really revolved around whatever my mom and stepdad wanted to do. We fit into *their* lives," she says. Today, evenings and weekends for many families find "one parent taking two kids this way and the other parent taking two kids that way. The family is on this hamster wheel of busy-ness." A hectic schedule teaches your kids how to *do,* but not necessarily how to simply *be.*

In addition, during the 70- or 80-something years you'll likely be alive, the time you spend raising your kids will probably account for only a small fraction. "If you're presently in this important phase, are you even able to enjoy it?" Dr. Solomon asks.

Also, are you developing as an individual during these years—and as a couple, with your spouse—so you'll be prepared for the rest of your life when you move on from the child-rearing portion?

Here's how to adjust your settings to find a good balance.

Establish values as a couple and family. You've already determined the values you want to follow as an individual. Now search for the ones that can guide you as a couple and as a family. Perhaps you'll put a premium on time together, showing your love for each other, honesty, good communication, living within your means, or doing your best.

Agree among yourselves which values will be most important within your home, Dr. Solomon suggests. These will then become a measuring tool of sorts, like a level with a little floating bubble. As you consider how your family will schedule its time, hold up each activity against these values. If they truly align, then by all means sign yourselves up for band, choir, martial arts, team sports, spelling bees, and tutoring sessions. But if activities don't measure up to your values, this tool will help you skip them without regret.

If you want to set goals that ensure you're living according to your values, Dr. Solomon suggests using *process* goals ("Are our choices and behaviors honoring our values?") rather than *outcome* goals ("Is Timmy getting all As?"). Process goals are within your control; outcome goals aren't necessarily.

Check in. Regularly touch base with the other stakeholders in your home to see how everyone's doing, Dr. Solomon says. You and your spouse might review once a year—perhaps on your anniversary—the degree to which your relationship is living up to your values. This could be a time to adjust your processes and provide feedback to each other.

You might also set up a weekly family meeting to discuss what's going well, who's struggling and needs help, and what the next week's schedule looks like.

Be present. Talk to each other. Spend time together. Make yourself available to your spouse and kids. "Being part of an intimate relationship and a family is ultimately about enjoying and nurturing the space in between people. These days, it's so darn easy to fill up the space in between people with whatever's on your phone. But life's meaning comes from being present for our important relationships. We're more connected than ever . . . but less present than ever," Dr. Solomon says.

This is the *being* that you might miss by continually *doing*. In some regards, it's easier to drive, drop off, pick up, and check off events from your calendar than to fill quiet time with meaningful interactions, Dr. Solomon says. Plus, you may feel out of step with other parents if you aren't hustling as hard as they are. But leave some of your time unscheduled.

During your time together, set limits on your digital devices to keep them from pulling you away from the present moment. Perhaps you'll turn them off during certain times of the day, or you'll set them in another room whenever you're having a conversation. Your marriage or partnership especially needs this time.

"Marriages are more fragile than parent-child relationships. In a marriage that goes days, weeks, or months without engaged presence, the bucket gets really empty. That sense of being emotionally disengaged from each other opens the door to all kinds of yucky stuff that can end up killing a marriage," Dr. Solomon says.

Keep acting like you're trying to win your spouse. You may be married, but proceed as if you're still dating, too, Dr. Solomon urges. That means:

- Setting aside one-on-one time with your spouse so you can focus on each other
- Coming up with interesting conversations and listening to the other person's input
- Striving to make a good impression on your spouse
- Putting forth effort
- Making your spouse a priority

"The bottom line is that people go into marriage with the assumption that love is all you need, without realizing that love is a verb that has to be embodied, practiced, and nurtured, and which requires time, energy, and intention. If couples rarely date, it's hard to ask the marriage to sustain that," says Dr. Solomon, the author of *Loving Bravely: 20 Lessons of Self-Discovery to Help You Get the Love You Want.*

Let your kids be individuals. Remember that even though your kids may look like you and share some of your interests, they're not clones of you, says Susan Newman, PhD, a social psychologist and author of more than a dozen parenting and relationship books.[5]

Let them contribute to creating a schedule that provides them with happiness and meaning. Watch for signs of stress or burnout—like mood changes and physical symptoms such as headaches and stomachaches—and be open to letting them take a break from an activity when necessary. (Even though that can be tough if you've already invested a lot of money and energy into it, she notes.)

Let yourself evolve as an individual, too. "Keep up your social connections. You don't want to become so isolated that your entire social world collapses," Dr. Newman says. Someday your kids won't need you so much, and you'll have time to resume your interest in, say, tennis. So why let your mastery of your hobbies slide? Why allow a void to form that you'll someday need to fill? If an activity is important to your identity or sense of meaning, find some time to stay involved in it.

Set aside ample time to maintain friendships, too. While friends are important in your middle years, they become *critical* to your well-being later in life, especially if your adult children scatter to distant homes or your spouse dies, Dr. Newman says.

"Your friends are people who can go with you to the emergency room, bring in your mail, and cook for you if you're not feeling well. I've been watching an older friend of mine whose children don't live anywhere near her. Her friends have become her lifeline!" she adds.

Balancing everyone's needs—yours, your spouse's, your kids'—during a busy time of your life is a tall order. That's yet another reason to deliberately assign your time and your attention to the different areas of your life, and to adjust your Personal Settings periodically as needed.

Spirituality and Religion: Using a "Ready-Made Framework"

The significance of religion in American life has steadily eroded in the past century.

Compared to the generation before the Baby Boomers (the technical term for them was the Silent Generation), subsequent waves of Americans have been increasingly less likely to pray daily, go to church weekly, believe in God, or feel that religion is very important in their lives. (Interestingly, the belief in hell has held pretty steady, at roughly 56 percent.)[6]

Still, most people claim some sort of religious affiliation. A Pew Research Center survey from 2014 estimated the US population as roughly 71 percent Christian, 2 percent Jewish, and less than 1 percent apiece Buddhist, Muslim, and Hindu. People with no religious identification—they're atheist, agnostic, or "nothing in particular"—weigh in at 23 percent.[7]

Though our beliefs are changing, religion and spirituality (which I'll refer to as "religion" for the sake of simplicity) can provide an important source of support for your sense of meaning, says Daryl Van Tongeren, PhD. He's an assistant professor of psychology at Hope College in Holland, Michigan, who has an interest in religion and meaning.[8]

"Religion or spirituality gives a ready-made framework or lens through which people can see the world. I think that's one way that religion appeals to a lot of people, by providing this worldview that helps make sense of the world," he says. "Religion also offers a community of like-minded individuals. When you're surrounded by people who can essentially validate what you believe, you find meaning by interacting with them and sharing moments that make life so special."

Of course, one's religion may also promise some sort of additional life after this one is over. "Religion kind of outsmarts death by saying, 'If you're right about religion, death isn't going to end all the meaning you have in this life.' It's like a path for meaning to continue into perpetuity or into eternity. I'd argue that the appeal that religion offers in the meaning landscape is this extension that death doesn't end all the great things about this life," he says.

I'm not here to tell you to adopt any religious conviction or change your customs. But if you already have a religious practice, it's not a bad idea to evaluate your approach toward it. Are you growing in your faith? Is your religion supporting your life's meaning? Or are you struggling, merely going through the motions, or in need of spiritual renewal? Consider these specific steps for getting more from your practice.

Explore the elements that provide meaning. Many major religions teach the importance of forgiveness, and this act may provide benefits now and at the end of your life. In 2015, Dr. Van Tongeren and colleagues conducted a study with 105 couples who were married or dating seriously. For 4 months, each participant wrote down "the most severe offense their partner had committed during the previous 2 weeks." Then they noted their level of forgiveness for their partner and how well their partner tried to make amends. Over time, those who regularly forgave reported greater meaning in life.[9]

"I'm a big believer that relationships are a huge source of meaning for many people, and fractures in relationships cause additional stress, pain, and negative emotion," he says. At the ends of their lives, many people ruminate on unresolved hurts between themselves and their loved ones. "I think mending those fences is going to play a large role in someday providing a sense of closure. It's going to repair relationships that are a pretty big source of meaning."

In the next chapter, you'll learn a process for offering forgiveness to others—and yourself.

Gratitude is another component that religions commonly emphasize. This means being aware of and thankful for the good things (or even the challenging things) in your life. Another of Dr. Van Tongeren's studies from 2015 found that people who wrote notes of gratitude felt a greater sense of meaning in their lives.[10]

Find gratitude rituals that appeal to you. Perhaps you can count the things for which you're grateful each night before bed or each morning when you wake up. Give thanks before you eat a meal. When you're annoyed, redirect your thoughts to something that's going *right*. When life gets hard, see if you can find benefits in this challenge, or a silver lining that deserves your thankfulness. Also, check out your religion's texts to see how they describe the value of gratitude.

Carry a sense of humility. It's possible to develop an intolerant "us versus them" outlook from one's religious practice, like the sense that other religions have it wrong or that their worshippers are going to be in for a surprise in the afterlife. Beware of this pitfall and try to steer away from such negative judgments.

"There's a certain way of being religious that provides people with security, but it can make you less agreeable or maybe less tolerant toward people who are different from you. On the other hand, if you're more oriented toward growth and expanding yourself, that's going to make you more tolerant, but it doesn't do the best job of providing you security. The trick is to find some type of middle ground," Dr. Van Tongeren says.

"If I were a betting person, I'd put my money on humility as a good way forward. Humility isn't necessarily saying, 'What I believe is wrong or my beliefs have no value,' but I think we can hold our religious beliefs with humility knowing that in the end we *could* be wrong, and knowing that we have a lot to learn from other people," he adds.

Other religions may be able to show you that they share essentials with your belief system (like forgiveness and gratitude). If your community offers interdenominational gatherings or open houses at different worship sites—or you know someone with a different faith—consider using this as an opportunity to enrich your point of view.

Talk to others in the know. Be ready to consult with a clergy member if you feel that your religious practice isn't providing the comfort you want to take from it, you're feeling guilty or anxious, or you simply want to grow in your faith. If others in your congregation are setting examples in their religious practices or personal lives that could serve as good models for you to follow, spend time talking with them. How do they derive meaning and happiness from their faith? What challenges have they worked through?

Research shows that religion can be a buffer against life's stresses and uncertainties. On the other hand, religion may also make you feel *worse* if you feel that God is angry with you or absent from your life; if you're not practicing religious observations correctly; or if you've committed actions or had thoughts that your religion says are sinful.[11] It may be helpful to discuss such feelings with a clergy member.

Death Helped Researcher Live More in the Moment

For Daryl Van Tongeren, PhD, whose research takes him to the intersection of death and religion, mortality isn't just an academic interest.

"Six years ago, when I was in graduate school, my brother died unexpectedly. He was 34 and had three kids under the age of 5, and he was a huge cheerleader for my research. Losing him made me rethink the assumptions I had in my life," he says. Namely, how he used his time.

"Instead of thinking that 'Being a good son, a good husband, or a good friend are all things I can work on in the future,' it shifted my focus to 'How do I do things in the present?' It's a more mindful approach. Since all we're guaranteed is now, what can I do to improve relationships now?" he says.

"Keeping an awareness of my mortality helps me take advantage of the moment and not assume things will always be there in the future—whether that's for my wife and I to take the trip we'd been putting off, fix things in our marriage we want to address, or be more intentional in our relationships."

Altruism: Good for Others, Good for You

In college, Sara Konrath began puzzling over a woman named Ruth, who appeared in her family's life when she was a child.[12]

Ruth volunteered with a nonprofit that helped single mothers. Konrath's mom was raising eight kids on her own, and she welcomed the helping hand.

"Ruth became a grandmother figure for us. She would take a few of us at a time to her beautiful country house and give our mom a break. After I got older, I was wondering more about her, since she didn't talk about *why* she did good; she just did it. It seemed very altruistic—which I define as 'focusing on the needs of others'—but I also saw that it brought her a lot of joy and satisfaction," she says.

Konrath's curiosity about why some people want to help others became her focus as she pursued a PhD in social psychology. She's now a researcher in the Lilly Family School of Philanthropy at Indiana University–Purdue University Indianapolis.

As you may recall from the previous section, many experts consider altruism to be an important component of a meaningful life. Of course, you *can* devote your life solely to fulfilling your own personal wants and needs. But if you consider that "meaning in life is gained, in part, from transcending the self and attaching to something outside of, or larger than, oneself," then altruistic actions can be one way to make that bigger connection, Dr. Van Tongeren wrote in a 2015 article.[13]

Evidence makes a pretty convincing case for altruism's ability to increase your physical and emotional well-being. Controlled research, in which one group of people was randomly chosen to volunteer and another group was asked to refrain, found that the volunteers had less depression and higher self-esteem, Dr. Konrath says. Research compiling the results of earlier studies also found that volunteering was linked with a 24 percent lower risk of dying in middle-aged and older adults![14]

However, not all altruistic gestures are created equal. And it's possible that service to others could leave you feeling *less* at ease with your life. Here's how to get the most good out of your do-gooding.

Focus on others rather than your own benefit. It's okay to get personal enjoyment from volunteering or making donations, to enjoy the warm feeling it provides, or the chance to be around good-hearted people. Just make sure those aren't your *only* reasons.

"My research suggests that if you're doing volunteer service or making donations because you're intending to get something back—even if it's something reasonable, like a tax refund or learning something new, or if you're using it as a stepping-stone to a new job—if that's your primary reason for doing it, it's not going to feel as satisfying to you," Dr. Konrath says.

In addition, your altruism may benefit your longevity less if you're doing it out of self-centered motivations. In one study, Dr. Konrath and colleagues found that people who volunteered, especially those who did it often, had an overall lower risk of dying. But the volunteers who said they served because of what *they* received from volunteering had a similar risk of dying as the nonvolunteers.[15]

Keep your eyes off the clock. It may be better to think about your commitment to serving others in terms of the amount of *attention* you give it, rather than *time*. "I don't like the idea of clocking in or checking something off a list. Rather than putting it into a planner, make it sort of a regular part of your mind-set," she says.

Take care of yourself, too. If you're running around volunteering so much that you're getting stressed out or are neglecting your own health, you may be overdoing it. Be sure to also honor your own needs for stillness and relaxation, Dr. Konrath says.

As with everything else, your service to others may need to be trimmed back if it's keeping you from reaching the goals you want to attain elsewhere in your life.

Share your beliefs with your family. If the notion of creating an impact that continues to "ripple" outward after you're gone inspires you, remember that service to others can create long-lasting waves. So why not multiply that ripple effect by instilling these values in the children in your life?

If you can bring your kids or grandkids along on your volunteer time, do so. (Not all sites have room for kids, especially young ones.) In your everyday life, teach them the value of giving to others, Dr. Konrath urges. "Kids need to learn from example. If you're making donations as part of your daily life, talk about why you do it. Like when you're going through clothes they've outgrown, say, 'Oh, we know a person who'd love these clothes. Let's take the best pieces to share.'"

Focus on the process, not the results. Do what you can for others, but let the outcome remain outside of your control. A person who's panhandling might use your money to buy cigarettes, so if it's vital to you that your $5 go toward necessities, perhaps you should donate to a homeless agency.

Also remember that even if you pour considerable energy and resources into helping an individual or family get on their feet, other powerful forces will also influence whether or not they achieve success, like their education, job history, mental health, substance use, opportunities, and so forth.

Dr. Konrath told me that as an adult, she was able to reconnect with Ruth. The older woman told her that not all the mothers and children she worked with years ago went on to flourish. Dr. Konrath thanked her mentor for improving her childhood at a time when "I didn't see too many positives in my life," and told Ruth how she helped launch her career in altruism research.

Because of the time and love Ruth shared, the ripple she started is still traveling outward.

Practice Can Boost Your Compassion for Others

Even in adulthood, it's possible to increase your capacity to care about strangers. In a 2013 study, researchers asked participants to practice "compassion training." During the sessions, a recording guided them to wish for joy, happiness, and freedom from suffering for a loved one. They repeated this sentiment toward themselves, a random acquaintance, an enemy, and the world in general.[16]

Later, when they played what they thought was an online game, those who practiced compassion training were more likely to share game money with another player who was being treated unfairly.

Give this a try! You can find an audio compassion training guide by searching online for the researcher's name—Helen Weng—along with "compassion meditation." It's also available online through the University of Wisconsin–Madison's Center for Healthy Minds.[17]

Practice Lifelong Self-Improvement

"Live as if you were going to die tomorrow; study as if you were to live forever," wrote the 15th-century Dutch scholar Desiderius Erasmus. (Cause of death: dysentery.)[18, 19]

The world is filled with so much wonderful knowledge to uncover, puzzles to decipher, and skills to master that you'll never finish all of it. But you can certainly try. And in the process, you might extend your brain's working life.

In an Australian study from 2016, researchers compared a group of older adults who took at least a year's worth of part-time college classes with a group who didn't advance their education. Over a 4-year period, those who went to school were more likely to have an increase in "cognitive reserve."[20] A brain with more cognitive reserve may be better able to continue functioning despite age- or disease-related changes.[21]

You may not have to seek formal classroom education to reap benefits from learning. A 2014 study following nearly 2,000 adults made a particularly compelling finding in the participants with a genetic variant that put them at higher risk of Alzheimer's. Among this group, cognitive problems began roughly 9 years later in people with "high lifetime intellectual enrichment." The researchers defined "intellectual enrichment" generously, such as reading newspapers and magazines, playing music, creating art, participating in a book club, and watching movies.[22]

As you're going about your daily activities, devote ample time to taking care of your mind. A wide buffet is available for feeding it, and you can do so fairly cheaply these days.

Sign up for a library card, and use it frequently. Watch challenging films with ambiguous conclusions. Listen to the music that your kids or grandkids are playing, and figure out the message of the lyrics. Go online to meetup.com and look for Meetup groups in your area that are gathering to discuss current events, speak foreign languages, talk about professional issues, or wrestle with intellectual and philosophical ideas.

While you're online, look up the term *MOOC*. This stands for "massive open online courses," which include a vast number of *free* classes created by prestigious universities. Or if you want to learn in an actual classroom setting, check your local colleges to see if they offer opportunities at a discount. (For example, you may be able to audit classes without receiving credit.)

As long as you're in possession of a mind, never let it starve.

Never let it grow complacent, sluggish, or bored.

Keep exposing it to unfamiliar situations. Maintain lofty expectations for its performance. Keep sharpening it, for it's a tool you might be wielding for a very long time.

Get Some of the Stuff That Feels Good: Physical Pleasures; Entertainment and Travel; and Acquiring Money and Possessions

In the Food Guide Pyramid that the federal government once used for illustrating a healthy diet, the little point at the top represented fats, oils, and sweets. You were advised to eat desserts, greasy fast food, and other guilty pleasures sparingly, as your occasional departure from the virtuous foods at the base of the pyramid.[23]

That said, without special treats sprinkled atop your more meaningful choices, that pyramid wouldn't be complete, would it? It certainly wouldn't reach its peak.

The same is true for life in general.

A well-rounded life provides room to have fun for fun's sake. You're not obliged to live completely in pursuit of noble goals; to serve others with no thought for your own needs; or to nurture only your spirit and ignore your flesh.

Physical pleasures can offer transcendent experiences that elevate you above your normal routine: the perfect morsel of food; the heady buzz of wine and conversation with friends; or the moment when your bare skin seems to become electrified upon contact with another's.

If your leisure time offers the chance to unwrap a foreign shore like a gift when you disembark from your ship, or to gaze in awe at a multimillion-dollar entertainment spectacle for a few hours, why wouldn't you? These moments may be among those you'll remember for the rest of your days.

For that matter, why *not* decorate your life with well-chosen possessions if you can afford to do so: the new car, nice home, good clothes, and shiny toys? Or, if you'd rather, why not acquire and invest money to assure a comfortable tomorrow for yourself and your loved ones? These earthly riches may be fleeting and temporary, but we can say the same about ourselves.

All of these pleasurable elements have their place in a life of meaning and enduring happiness. It's up to you to incorporate them in the right amounts so they remain balanced with your other pursuits.

As you indulge in physical pleasures, entertainment, or possessions, I'd recommend pausing periodically to ask yourself a few questions.

- **Am I going for quality or quantity?** Am I truly tasting this food? Am I paying attention to this bodily pleasure that I agreed to experience? Will I remember this moment in a month? A week? Even tomorrow? Is this the real thing—or just filler? *Mindfulness,* a quality we'll discuss in the next chapter, can enhance your awareness of and appreciation for these moments.

- **Am I enjoying this activity or possession for its own sake?** Or am I using this activity or this purchase to distract myself from some problem or to numb myself from some type of distress? Am I traveling *to* somewhere or fleeing *from* somewhere?

- **Could this cause unintended consequences?** Over time, could my choices be harmful to my physical or emotional health? Could they sicken or kill me early? Could this use of my time and money damage the legacy I want to leave behind? Am I so devoted to passing pleasures that I'm cutting into my limited time to cultivate meaning or lasting happiness?

- **Is anyone benefiting from this?** Am I sharing these experiences with friends or loved ones who'll remember them with me later? In these moments, am I making investments that will add up to something bigger—or am I just spilling valuable time into the gutter?

"I'm in the unique position where I can answer many people's question, 'Do you reap what you sow?' I see the reaping later in life," says Marc Agronin, MD, a Miami psychiatrist and author who works with seniors. "At the end of the day, what makes a difference is the depth of relationships one has with family and friends, community institutions and organizations, and the church, temple, synagogue, or mosque. I work with people rich and poor. Happiness in life, when they say you can't buy it, it's very true."

If you maintain an optimal balance as you divide your time, focus, and resources across these eight categories, you're going to go a long way toward living well (and setting yourself up for a happy death).

But your Personal Settings exercises offers more elements to adjust. After you do the exercises that follow, the next chapter will show you four factors you can fine-tune to bring more peace of mind about three phases of life that may continually challenge your well-being.

LIVE WELL, DIE HAPPY EXERCISES
Chapter 4

Welcome to your first of three Personal Settings pages. (See ends of Chapter 4, 5, and 6.) Please fill out the information here to describe your life right now. Return to these pages periodically to make adjustments as your priorities shift and your goals change or are met.

Work

MY CURRENT TIME/FOCUS INVESTMENT:

10%	20%	30%	40%	50%	60%	70%	80%	90%	100%

What are my long-term (5-year) goals for my work life? _____

_____

_____

What are my short-term (1-year) goals that will help me meet my long-term goals?

_____

_____

Am I spending enough time here to meet my goals? _____

Am I currently using my time well in terms of meeting my short- and long-term goals in this area? _____

If necessary, how should I adjust the amount of time I invest—or how I use it—to increase the odds that I'll meet my goals in this area? _____

_____

_____

Is the amount of time I'm spending in this area, or the way I'm spending it, causing any of the seven other uses of my life to suffer? _____

If yes, what adjustments could I make to fix it? _____

_____

_____

Religious/Spiritual Practice

MY CURRENT TIME/FOCUS INVESTMENT:

10%	20%	30%	40%	50%	60%	70%	80%	90%	100%

What are my long-term (5-year) goals for my religious or spiritual practice? _____

_____

What are my short-term (1-year) goals that will help me meet my long-term goals?

_____

Am I spending enough time here to meet my goals? _____

Am I currently using my time well in terms of meeting my short- and long-term goals in this area? _____

If necessary, how should I adjust the amount of time I invest—or how I use it—to increase the odds that I'll meet my goals in this area? _____

_____

Is the amount of time I'm spending in this area, or the way I'm spending it, causing any of the seven other uses of my life to suffer? _____

If yes, what adjustments could I make to fix it? _____

_____

Relationships with Spouse/Partner/Kids/ Other Family/Close Friends

MY CURRENT TIME/FOCUS INVESTMENT:

10%	20%	30%	40%	50%	60%	70%	80%	90%	100%

What are the values guiding my relationship with my spouse/partner? _____

_____

What are the values guiding my relationship with my kids? _____

_____

What are the values guiding my other important relationships? _____

_____

Am I currently using my time well in terms of living up to my values in these areas?

_____

If necessary, how should I adjust the amount of time I invest—or how I use it—so I'm living according to my important values? _____

_____

Is the amount of time I'm spending here, or the way I'm spending it, causing any of the seven other uses of my life to suffer? _____

If yes, what adjustments could I make to fix it? _____

_____

Altruism

MY CURRENT TIME/FOCUS INVESTMENT:

10%	20%	30%	40%	50%	60%	70%	80%	90%	100%

What are some motivations that fuel my interest in helping others? _____

_____

What are my goals for serving others? _____

_____

How can I serve others in a way that best adds to the legacy I wish to leave behind? _____

Am I spending enough time here to meet my goals? _____

Am I currently using my time well in terms of meeting my goals in this area? _____

_____

If necessary, how should I adjust the amount of time I invest—or how I use it—to increase the odds that I'll meet my goals in this area? _____

_____

Is the amount of time I'm spending in this area, or the way I'm spending it, causing any of the seven other uses of my life to suffer? _____

If yes, what adjustments could I make to fix it? _____

_____

_____

_____

Self-Improvement/Learning

MY CURRENT TIME/FOCUS INVESTMENT:

10%	20%	30%	40%	50%	60%	70%	80%	90%	100%

What are my long-term (5-year) goals for my intellectual development? _____

_____

_____

What are my short-term (1-year) goals that will help me meet my long-term goals?

Am I spending enough time here to meet my goals? _____

Am I currently using my time well in terms of meeting my short- and long-term goals in this area? _____

If necessary, how should I adjust the amount of time I invest—or how I use it—to increase the odds that I'll meet my goals in this area? _____

_____

_____

Is the amount of time I'm spending in this area, or the way I'm spending it, causing any of the seven other uses of my life to suffer? _____

If yes, what adjustments could I make to fix it? _____

_____

_____

_____

Place a dot on each gauge to indicate how you'd describe the general role that physical pleasure, entertainment and travel, and acquiring money and possessions play in your life.

PHYSICAL PLEASURE (eating, drinking, sex, various vices)	ENTERTAINMENT AND TRAVEL	ACQUIRING MONEY AND POSSESSIONS
Quality	Quality	Quality
Quantity	Quantity	Quantity
Doing it because it's enjoyable	Doing it because it's enjoyable	Doing it because it's enjoyable
Doing it as a distraction	Doing it as a distraction	Doing it as a distraction
No harmful/ unintended consequences	No harmful/ unintended consequences	No harmful/ unintended consequences
Likely harmful/ unintended	Likely harmful/ unintended	Likely harmful/ unintended
This has enduring benefits for me and others	This has enduring benefits for me and others	This has enduring benefits for me and others
This benefits only me temporarily	This benefits only me temporarily	This benefits only me temporarily

Change Your Perspective on the Past, Present, and Future

If time feels like it's moving faster than it did when you were a kid, you're not alone. Researchers have found that it's common in adulthood to get the sense that your life has picked up speed.[1]

Several theories might explain why time seems to move more briskly later in life, according to the *Scientific American* blog. For starters, each additional year represents a smaller chunk of the life you've lived so far. When you were 9, the coming year added another 11 percent to your life—quite a generous addition. At 59, the next year adds just 1.7 percent more—a thin sliver compared to what you've already experienced.

Also, you frequently encounter novel and memorable experiences in the time leading up to your early adulthood, like your first relationship; first job; graduations; and legal permission to drive, join the military, drink, and vote. After that, the landscape tends to present fewer milestones that feel so momentous. And later in life, when you're working, raising kids, and perhaps caring for parents, time may feel fleeting because you never seem to have enough of it.

Time is tricky. When you try to view it clearly, it can resist your efforts.

This chapter will help you adjust your focus on this sometimes distressing dimension of your life. Specifically, you'll learn how to better handle the three phases of time that will always be with you until your last breath.

Your past. As you grow older, more of it trails behind you. The past can become heavier if you pull an increasing load of loss, resentment, irritation, and guilt. Are you still unhappy that someone wronged you? Ashamed over an error that you feel *you* committed? These things add to the burden of the past.

Your present. You are here. Are you content with your career accomplishments? Did you pick the right spouse? Are you satisfied that when you had the choice of two doors to enter, you opened the correct one? Or have you fallen short of where you wanted to be? Are you struggling against your present circumstances? Do you stare at the ceiling in the dark, asking, "What if?"

Your future. You're racing into an unwritten mystery. Though you may have an expectation of what it will bring, invariably the future will surprise you. Perhaps it will offer great rewards and wash away the troubles in your life. Or the opposite could occur.

It's time to make a few adjustments. Each will allow you to turn up the intensity of a particular feature within your outlook. When you amplify these attitudes, you can:

- Reduce the burdens you carry from the past
- Experience greater satisfaction and joy from the current moment
- Anticipate the future with less unease—and more wonder

You've already used a significant portion of your life, perhaps even the majority. The rest may seem to pass even more swiftly. Adjusting these four settings will help ensure that you write the happiest, most meaningful life story possible in the remaining time available.

Setting 1: Forgiveness to Reduce the Burden of the *Past*

In 1990, psychologist Everett Worthington, PhD, turned his professional focus to the concept of forgiveness. In the following years, as the Virginia

Commonwealth University professor absorbed one jarring loss after another, his need to forgive became personal.[2]

First of all, his mother was murdered in the family home in 1995. For a day, Dr. Worthington's fury raged. Then he worked through the five steps in the program he'd developed to teach others to forgive. It's not in his basic nature to do so; he told the *Atlantic* magazine that after receiving a B on a paper from a college professor, he needed "10 years and a religious experience to forgive that guy."[3] But he was able to forgive the killer. (No one was ever convicted for the crime.)

A decade later, while traveling in Europe, he learned that his brother had taken his own life. Forgiving himself for the guilt he felt—perhaps he could have seen the signs or taken action to rescue his brother—was not easy.

"It took 3 years to get past that. It was not a very happy time," he says, pausing to chuckle. "That's the nicest thing I can say about that time." How would his life have proceeded had he not given himself forgiveness? "If I had lived with that for 10 to 15 years instead of 3, it would have been a pretty negative existence. I'm glad that God gave me an ability to forgive and to move forward and not stay mired in rumination."

A 2016 study found that young adults who'd experienced severe stress throughout their lives had poorer physical and mental health. So did those who offered forgiveness less frequently. But the harmful effect of stress on mental health was lessened in the people who showed more forgiveness.[4] That same year, British researchers who compiled the results of earlier studies found that people who attended forgiveness-based therapy after experiencing violence or other distress had less depression, anger, and stress.[5]

In research with families of patients in hospice, Dr. Worthington and colleagues found that only about 15 percent spoke of still needing to offer or request forgiveness. "It's certainly important for that 15 percent, but it's not universal. Many people have taken care of those issues early on instead of letting them sit until they're on their deathbed," he says. "Certainly it frees you up to deal with other things at the last minute."

This research also found that families of hospice patients were more likely to report depression if they were still carrying unresolved hurt, or if they felt that forgiveness was important but it hadn't been fully expressed.[6]

Has someone committed a wrong against you that you're still carrying as a grudge? Is a long-ago mistake still making you feel bad today? Now is the time to clean your slate and leave this unresolved pain in the past.

Do more than just "let it go." You have many options for dealing with injustice, Dr. Worthington says. At one end of the scale, you could choose revenge. A more middle-of-the-road approach—"letting go and moving on"—might sound healthier. But you can do even better.

"Just letting it go" merely relieves you of a negative, which is indeed a good thing. But taking the next step and moving into the territory of forgiving creates a positive feeling, he says. "Imagine having a relationship where you've been hurt in the past but saying, 'I've faced this and forgiven this. Can you forgive me for times I've messed up?' What a difference in the relationship that's going to make compared to, 'I'm moving on; I'm not going to worry about this anymore.'"

Psychologist Barbara Fredrickson, PhD, who led the study discussed on page 45 linking hedonic pleasures with gene expression associated with inflammation, developed the so-called broaden-and-build theory about positive emotions such as joy, contentment, and love. These emotions expand your palette of thoughts and actions. Over time, you develop more varied physical, mental, psychological, and social resources to draw upon when you face challenges. In contrast, *negative* emotions generate a narrow range of thoughts and actions, like whether to fight your threat or flee from it. Negative emotions encourage you to shrink your focus.[7, 8]

"If you've changed your emotion toward somebody to, 'I've forgiven them, and I've gone on and I feel better about them,' that creates that broaden-and-build cascade of positive emotions Fredrickson talks about," Dr. Worthington says.

Do you want a small and fearful life? Or a big, overflowing life that transcends the old ways of thinking that once hemmed you in? Forgiveness can help direct you toward the latter.

Understand what forgiveness is and isn't. One commonly accepted definition of forgiveness is: "a conscious, deliberate decision to release feelings of resentment or vengeance toward a person or group who has harmed you, regardless of whether they actually deserve your forgiveness."[9]

Forgiving doesn't mean you have to continue a marriage or maintain a friendship with someone, Dr. Worthington says. You don't have to leave yourself vulnerable to future harm. You can also hope someone receives justice for a crime he committed against you while offering him forgiveness.

Forgiveness also comes in two forms. *Decisional* forgiveness involves making a choice to not show anger or resentment toward this person. It's more of an intention about how you'll act later. *Emotional* forgiveness means replacing negative feelings with positive ones. According to Dr. Worthington, though decisional forgiveness is sometimes better for helping relationships heal, the emotional form of forgiveness provides more benefits for your health and well-being.[10]

REACH to forgive others. The following five-step forgiveness process that Dr. Worthington devised follows the acronym REACH.

Recreate the hurt that someone inflicted on you. Replay the story in your mind. Re-create it in detail, and picture how you responded to the experience. Now watch the event again, but this time try to see it from the perspective of a neutral observer, without a villain and a victim in the story.

Empathize with the person who hurt you. Think about when *you've* hurt other people. Did you do so while still having good intentions, or at least not the intention to cause harm? Is it possible to imagine that this person didn't mean to cause the degree of hurt you felt? Can you find compassion or empathy for this fellow imperfect human?

Give an **A**ltruistic gift of forgiveness. Think about times when others have offered you forgiveness, or you would have appreciated them granting it. Now pass this gift along. Helping others, without concern for our own benefit (in other words, altruism), is an important component of living well and dying happy. Here's a chance for you to share a kindness that benefits others *and* yourself.

Commit to it. Dr. Worthington suggests that you write out the forgiveness in a note that only you'll see, to make it feel more real. Date your note, list the person by name, and write down the offense you're forgiving.

Hold on to your forgiveness. Plan ahead for how you'll behave when you see this person again, he suggests. What could you do to display a pleasant demeanor if you feel angry in that moment? Also, keep in mind that if you do feel anger, fear, or sadness deep inside when you see this person again, it doesn't necessarily mean your forgiveness didn't stick; it could be that your brain is trying to protect you from being harmed again.

Forgive yourself, too. The process is similar when you forgive yourself for your own thoughts or actions. As Dr. Worthington describes in his book *Moving Forward,* you still recall, give an altruistic gift, commit, and hold on to the forgiveness. But here you examine your *own* offenses and offer the forgiveness to yourself. Also, the E stands for "**E**motionally replace unforgiveness with empathy." Be kind to yourself. Allow yourself to be imperfect, just as you understand when others fall short of the ideal.[11]

Take note: If you've harmed others, your work is not finished just because you've forgiven yourself, Dr. Worthington warns. You'll also need to make

---

Watch for This Warning Signal

How do you know when it's time to offer forgiveness? One sign is *rumination,* says psychologist Everett Worthington, PhD. This means you're repeatedly bringing up an offense, slight, or mistake from the past to chew upon again.

Rumination comes in several flavors, he says.

The angry type. You want to get even with the offender.

The anxious type. After suffering a hurt, you're worried that you'll be hurt again. You might start avoiding situations where you'll encounter this person, like skipping work meetings to stay away from a critical coworker.

The depressive type. You feel that you're hopelessly stuck in the situation that makes you feel bad.

Whichever type of rumination is at play, offering forgiveness— either to another person or to yourself—may help relieve this cycle, Dr. Worthington says.

---

amends. That may mean apologizing and trying to make right any damage you've caused (or paying some goodness forward into the world if the person you've harmed is avoiding you).

Adopt other qualities that go hand in hand with forgiveness. You can cultivate other characteristics that will help you spend less time stewing on past disappointments, Dr. Worthington says. These include *agreeableness,* which protects you from becoming offended as easily; *gratitude,* which helps keep your focus on the good parts of your life; and *humility,* which acknowledges that you have shortcomings, too.

These qualities aren't necessarily easy to acquire, but they're worth the effort.

Setting 2 and Setting 3: Mindfulness and Acceptance to Increase Your *Present* Well-Being

If you don't tend to your mind, it may wander away for a significant portion of your life.

Your attention drifts to the past, perhaps replaying a highlight of joy, but often nursing an argument, lamenting a missed opportunity, or yearning for a vanished piece of your life that can never return. Or it leaps ahead of you to imagine some future dreadfulness: the lost job, the collapsed marriage, the accidental tragedy.

Meanwhile, you carry the misguided notion that you can control vast swaths of your surroundings that are actually well outside your jurisdiction.

Want to bring your attention back to the here and now? Try some *mindfulness.* Want to stop struggling against burdens you don't even need to be lifting? Develop *acceptance.*

These assets work well together to improve the present moment, say Kirk Strosahl, PhD, and Patricia Robinson, PhD. They're prominent psychologists within a field of psychotherapy called Acceptance and Commitment Therapy (ACT). The two have coauthored a number of books on applying the principles of ACT to your daily life, and they spoke with me while taking a break from writing another.

Mindfulness is a concept borrowed from Buddhism that's become a mainstream approach to relieving anxiety and depression and improving emotional well-being. When you're mindful, you're continually paying attention to:

- What's happening around you in *the real world*
- The thoughts arising in your *mind*
- The sensations in your *body*

The idea is to observe this information without judgment. Also, your mind stays focused on the here and now, instead of getting swept away into the past or future.[12]

Acceptance means accepting events and situations you can't control. But it goes deeper. "It's turning toward painful feelings, thoughts, evaluations, memories, changes in your body, and aches and pains, and letting them be there without evaluation or struggle," Dr. Strosahl says.

Someone with a low level of acceptance "would be a person who's more guided by rules about how life should be and how people should act," Dr. Robinson says. Invariably, the real world doesn't follow your rules, and if you won't accept that, disappointment ensues.

"I think you see a lot of people stuck in that kind of right and wrong thinking, and probably missing out on the moment-to-moment joys of everyday life," she says.

To appreciate the present moment more fully, here's how to adjust your mindfulness and acceptance settings.

Improve your vocabulary. Often, people have trouble putting their finger on exactly how they're reacting to events around them, Dr. Strosahl says. How are they feeling? Who knows—they can't even find the words to describe it! To better define where you're currently standing, expand your emotional dictionary.

Do you have a vague sense of dissatisfaction in your life, perhaps related to a career choice? Take a closer look and try to describe more accurately how you're feeling. Is an emotion bothering you—maybe worry over your kids' college funds? Do you have a physical sensation, like a churning stomach? Is a memory nagging at you, maybe an uncle's prediction that your business wouldn't thrive? "What words are you going to put to that? Forming a description helps you create a road map of your internal world.

"Learning to use words to describe how you feel is sometimes called *affect labeling,* and it is regarded as a key part of learning to understand, integrate, and regulate emotional experience. It keeps your nervous system in check so that you don't overreact to emotions in the moment," Dr. Strosahl says.

Wash your hands. ACT teaches that there's a difference between "clean" and "dirty" suffering. Learning to distinguish between the two can help you live a life with less struggle.

"Your body will gradually break down. Maybe your spouse will die before you. Maybe you'll lose a child before you pass away, like my mom did. That's the *clean* stuff. That's the contract you signed when you were born," he says.

"The *dirty* stuff is the feelings you generate when you refuse to accept the clean stuff. Now you get all the additional suffering that comes along with refusing to accept the fact that, say, your son is in prison. You don't let yourself think about it, and when you do, you break down in tears, and you feel humiliated around people at church. Clean suffering is inevitable. Dirty suffering is completely avoidable."

If this brings to mind asking for serenity to accept things you can't change, courage to change the things you can, and wisdom to know the difference, you're on to something. Dr. Strosahl says ACT is "the walking, talking Serenity Prayer."

Follow the Golden Rule . . . with a twist. While we're finding contemporary uses for adages that Grandma once cross-stitched, here's another: Do unto yourself as you should do unto others. In short, be self-compassionate. Treat yourself every bit as kindly as you would, say, a friend with a painful illness, Dr. Strosahl advises.

Remember that you have flaws, just as everyone else does. Your life has fallen short of the heights that you once strived for, just like everyone else's. You have failed, just like everyone else has, he says. Accept your shortcomings, just as you strive to accept them in others.

Acknowledge your connections. A common source of pain is the notion that you shouldn't have to face change and loss because you're somehow separate or different from everyone else, Dr. Strosahl says. But you're not separate; you're interconnected with all of humanity. This teaching comes from Buddhism. (This warning arises again later in the book—it's something you may want to remember if you're ever seeking a miraculous cure for a serious health problem.)

Now is always a good time to start accepting unwanted changes. As our discussion has repeatedly made clear, practicing now can help you better cope with the final change waiting at the end of your life. "Kirk's mother, in her last years, would have periods when she would stop breathing," Dr. Robinson says. "She described them as 'practicing for death.' She wasn't afraid when she said that. She was *curious*. That embodies what we're talking about."

Turn off your cruise control. Finally, as you go about your daily schedule, avoid using your autopilot, Dr. Strosahl says.

"Being intentional is really the antidote for living on autopilot. It allows you to make choices based upon your values rather than just obeying social norms and expectations that produce no sense of life vitality, meaning, or purpose. Living with intention brings you into the moment and puts you into contact with what really matters to you," he says.

So pay attention. Focus on what people are saying rather than the response you're going to give. Assume less. Avoid automatic reactions. Strive to live in the real, actual world that surrounds you, rather than the world that exists only in your mind. This is what it means to be mindful.

Setting 4: Tolerate More Uncertainty for an Enjoyable *Future*

In the 2013 animated movie *The Croods,* a prehistoric family reacts differently to unfamiliar situations. The father retreats in fear from uncertainty. But his teenage daughter's curiosity spurs her to fearlessly embrace the unusual.

If too many of our ancient ancestors had approached uncertainty at either extreme—trembling in their caves until they starved or naively approaching vicious animals to pet them—humanity might not have survived, says

Dying Doctor and His Wife
Faced the End with Mindfulness

"You die like you live," says Julie Chippendale. Her husband, Thomas, died as the couple had lived: mindfully.[13]

In 1994, they attended a course on Mindfulness-Based Stress Reduction taught by Jon Kabat-Zinn, PhD, professor emeritus at the University of Massachusetts, who pioneered the practice of mindfulness for physical and mental well-being.

"What he was talking about blew us away. It was so simple yet so profound," she says. A nurse by training, Julie says she was always interested in "healing rather than curing." Tom—a neurologist who surfed, wrote poetry, and collected six academic degrees—found that mindfulness fit well with his interest in holistic medicine.

After he was diagnosed with lung cancer in July 2013, "he knew he most likely didn't have long to live," Julie says. "Most people would be so scared of the diagnosis that they'd do the first thing their doctor said to do. But the way we lived our lives before that diagnosis informed every step."

To be mindful is to be aware of events in your surroundings, your body, and your mind without automatic judgment. So, Julie says, "we

Nicholas Carleton, PhD, associate professor of psychology at the University of Regina, Canada.[14]

Most of us have a moderate fear of the unknown (or a related idea, intolerance of uncertainty), he says. All things being equal, humans don't generally *like* the unknown, he says, but we cope with it okay.

Dr. Carleton and other researchers have found that people with anxiety disorders such as generalized anxiety and obsessive-compulsive disorder, and also depression, tend to have higher levels of intolerance of uncertainty.[15]

He suspects that humanity is forgetting how to cope with the mysterious unknown, due largely to wireless devices. "If I want to find my wife right now were not reacting from a fear of, 'Oh no, we have to get rid of this.'"

After a month of exploring his options, Tom began chemotherapy, which seemed to halt the disease. But eventually it spread. He stopped treatment and turned his attention to his closest relationships. The Chippendales' adult children moved home for 3 months, and the couple would invite friends over, asking them to tell Tom anything that was on their minds.

Until he died suddenly of a blood clot, Tom created beautiful drawings that quoted sayings and poems he found meaningful. On one he wrote the Buddha's Five Remembrances. In part, this teaching reminds us that our nature is to grow old, grow sick, and die, and we will someday be separated from all that we hold dear. This is the reality of impermanence.

"Mindfulness practice is paying attention to the reality of life and death. When someone dies, you stop, let it in, and feel it, instead of moving on to the next thing in this culture, whether it's having a drink, going shopping, or staying busy," says Julie, who continues to teach mindfulness and yoga.

"You have to practice mindfulness every day. Then when someone's dying, it's just another moment."

and be sure she's safe, I can do that in 2 seconds! We're losing the opportunity to practice not knowing and being okay with that. We're losing the opportunity to practice being uncertain, because we have access to Google and feel like it answers all our questions," he says.

Right now, as we stand in the present moment, we have our entire past at our backs. It's familiar; we mostly remember what it contains. But the future that we'll step into in the next moment is completely uncertain, totally unknown. We have expectations for what it will bring us and how we'll respond. But we can't truly know for sure, can we?

That uncertainty and unknown will be in front of you until your final moment. Take a look at whether you want to adjust how you'll cope with it. If you suspect you're dialed more to "shrinking in dread" than "cautiously enthusiastic," here's how to fine-tune your life's settings to a more comfortable level.

Take the quiz. A 12-question tool that Dr. Carleton helped develop, the Intolerance of Uncertainty Scale—Short Form, can show you how confident you feel about what's around the next corner. Ready?[16]

The Intolerance of Uncertainty Scale—Short Form

	Not at all characteristic of me	A little characteristic of me	Somewhat characteristic of me	Very characteristic of me	Entirely characteristic of me
1. Unforeseen events upset me greatly.	1	2	3	4	5
2. It frustrates me not having all the information I need.	1	2	3	4	5
3. Uncertainty keeps me from living a full life.	1	2	3	4	5
4. One should always look ahead so as to avoid surprises.	1	2	3	4	5
5. A small unforeseen event can spoil everything, even with the best of planning.	1	2	3	4	5
6. When it's time to act, uncertainty paralyzes me.	1	2	3	4	5
7. When I am uncertain, I can't function very well.	1	2	3	4	5
8. I always want to know what the future has in store for me.	1	2	3	4	5
9. I can't stand being taken by surprise.	1	2	3	4	5
10. The smallest doubt can stop me from acting.	1	2	3	4	5
11. I should be able to organize everything in advance.	1	2	3	4	5
12. I must get away from all uncertain situations.	1	2	3	4	5

Reprinted from the *Journal of Anxiety Disorders*, 21/1, RN Carleton, PJ Norton, GJG Asmundson, Fearing the Unknown: A Short Version of the Intolerance of Uncertainty Scale, 105-117, 2007, with permission from Elsevier.

Your score can range from 12 to 60. In a 2012 study, a national sample of adults scored around 30 on average. So, if your score is roughly 20 to 30, your intolerance of uncertainty is likely not causing you problems, Dr. Carleton says.[17]

In that study, groups of people with social anxiety, panic, general anxiety, obsessive-compulsive, or major depressive disorders scored an average of 37 to 43. If your score is 35 to 40 or higher, it may be time to take a look—on your own or with a mental health professional—at whether your need for certainty is so rigid that it's related to other concerns, such as anxiety or depression, he says.

Get some help. If you do decide to visit a mental health professional to discuss intolerance of uncertainty, the time you spend working on your issues may lead to several important benefits. In a 2013 study, more than 30 adults with an anxiety disorder (many of whom also had depression) participated in up to 18 sessions of cognitive behavioral therapy.[18]

In this process, people work with a therapist to "uncover unhealthy patterns of thought and how they may be causing self-destructive behaviors and beliefs. By addressing these patterns, you develop constructive ways of thinking that will produce healthier behaviors and beliefs," according to the National Alliance on Mental Illness.[19]

After the treatment, participants had a significant drop in their intolerance for uncertainty. Those who saw more progress also had greater improvement in their anxiety and depression symptoms.

Choose not to know. The next time you're pondering a minor mystery, leave your phone in your pocket. Refrain from Googling. Allow yourself to experience the uncertainty that is becoming so unfamiliar in the 21st century.

"Let's say we're having a couple of pints and debating whether Chicago or New York is bigger," Dr. Carleton says. (As an American, this is not a mystery to me. But I have no clue about Ontario and Quebec.) "Rather than whipping out the cell phone to find out, why not *not*? Why not leave the phone out of it? Do you really need to know this second?"

Are you struggling to remember the name of the character actor in the

Former Pro Cyclist Shows How to Stay Balanced through Health Changes

The first stage of the women's 1991 Tour de France began, and cyclist Maureen Manley took off. The event might have been yet another highlight on her way to the next year's Olympics.

Even as a kid, she'd pedaled the streets of her neighborhood imagining crowds cheering her on. She later joined the women's US cycling team, winning awards in national and world championships.

But recently her eyesight had become blurry. And on this day's race, she lost her vision entirely, flew off the road, and crashed. A diagnosis of multiple sclerosis abruptly ended her cycling career at age 26.

Now a speaker, wellness consultant, and life coach who lives with a condition that can cause a variety of disabling symptoms, Manley understands the health changes that nearly *all* of us will encounter if we live long enough. Here's her take on how to deal with physical losses, unwanted detours in your life's path, and an uncertain future.

Find other activities that reflect your passions. "My soul is a cyclist. It's in my DNA," Manley says. Her life as an athlete provided camaraderie with her team and helped her explore her abilities and express her passion.

When professional cycling disappeared as a career option, she explored new opportunities to fuel her meaning and happiness. (She still rides, though not at a world-class level.) "I had to lean into things that brought joy in other ways," she says. As you learned earlier, you can use many strategies to support your life's mission. When one is no longer possible, how can you pursue your mission in a different way?

Make good use of your time off the grid. Manley calls the adaptation period after a jolting change, like the diagnosis of a serious illness, "the wilderness." You may feel stunned, knocked off your feet,

movie you're watching? Stifle the urge to pull up the Internet Movie Database, and let your brain find the answer on its own. Want to check your e-mail inbox because you're bored? Try *not* checking it for 30 minutes. "We have a million years' worth of humans who lived without cell phones. But when you and hopeless. Some people just set up camp in the wilderness "and make that their story," she says. Devise a plan to get out of the wilderness, but choose your path with care.

First, resist the urge to grab at solutions. "Our culture is so used to having fixes for things. But we're not used to adapting to them," she says. Take a breath. Be loving and kind to yourself. Give yourself some time just to *be* with this development, rather than frantically *doing* something to fix it.

Absorb wisdom from people who have already figured out this challenge. "Having a mentor is a great thing," she says. Find an encouraging role model who's living a meaningful life despite the type of challenge you've encountered. One possible source of such mentors might be a support group. Look for a group that uses its time to support each other in solutions, rather than just focusing on the difficulty of the problem.

Know the difference between technical and adaptive challenges. Chronic health conditions can present two types of difficulty. One is *technical,* which requires you to figure out what to do about it; in Manley's case, that meant seeking the best treatments for her MS. Too many people stop there and don't work on the other challenge, which is *adaptive,* she says. In her case, that meant finding out how to not just cope with MS, but to *thrive* with it.

Technical challenges require knowledge that you obtain from outside sources. Adaptive challenges require you to develop your own wisdom, she explains. If she'd merely tried to "fix" the technical challenges of her MS, she'd still be sitting in that camp out in the middle of the wilderness, she says. "This is how I've done well in my life. It's my ability to be with the MS and work with what still functions well that allows me to do what I do."

tell people to do this stuff, you can see them become more fearful in front of you because you're taking away their certainty," Dr. Carleton says.

Conversely, learn more about important mysteries. "If you're anxious about something and you don't want to be, go meet it, learn about it, and interact with it, whatever *it* is, assuming it's safe," Dr. Carleton says. "I am a little afraid of sharks, and I'm not interested in diving into shark-infested water. But if I'm scared of dying or scared of getting older, then I should go talk to seniors. They've got a *way* better perspective on it than I do."

By spending time with the elderly—and people who are approaching the end of life, for that matter—you can receive valuable lessons and cautionary tales that help you plot a satisfying and rewarding course into your unwritten future.

Like with the recurring advice about phones, this isn't the last time you'll read about visiting with older people or individuals who are dying, by the way. That much is certain.

LIVE WELL, DIE HAPPY EXERCISES
Chapter 5

Let's adjust a few more personal settings. Work through these exercises now, and return to them regularly to refresh your levels of forgiveness, mindfulness, acceptance, and the ability to tolerate uncertainty.

Has my mind recently been ruminating on an event or situation in which someone embarrassed, harmed, or offended me?

Yes	No

If so, might I feel better if I worked through the process of forgiving this person?

Yes	No

Has my mind recently been ruminating on an event or situation in which I embarrassed, harmed, or offended someone else?

Yes	No

If so, would I feel better if I worked through the process of forgiving myself for this situation?

Yes	No

How could I also make amends to this person for what I did? _____

_____

_____

_____

_____

_____

Over the past 24 hours, how mindful and attentive was I toward the world unfolding around me, as opposed to being fully immersed in my thoughts and running on autopilot?

Mindful and attentive   **Fully lost in my thoughts/on autopilot**

Think of some important worries that are currently demanding your time and attention. Write them down on the chart below grouping them by whether you *can* or *can't* fully control them.

Then, take a look at your list. Cross off any item that you find easy to accept. What's left is your homework. In your "can control" list, come up with ways to change the situation from a negative to a positive. In the "can't control" list, consider ways you can move from nonacceptance toward acceptance.

What I Can Control	What I Can't Control
1.	
2.	
3.	
4.	
5.	
6.	
7.	
8.	
9.	
10.	

How long can I currently go without looking up information (e.g., e-mail, weather maps, directions, store hours) on my digital device when I have a nonurgent desire to know it?

I can look it up later or not at all   **I need to look it up immediately**

CHAPTER 6

Keep Adjusting as Your Body Changes

Six years ago, yet another patient limped into the office to see Elizabeth Eckstrom, MD, MPH, with health problems that seemed age-related, but weren't necessarily so.[1]

"I first met him when he was about 71. He was a nice guy, highly educated, with a very successful life. But he was barely able to walk, and he was in terrible pain and quite depressed," says Dr. Eckstrom, the director of geriatrics at Oregon Health and Science University in Portland.

"He was typical of a lot of older patients: They start to have some arthritis or back pain and get into a cycle of decreased exercise, taking pain pills, getting more depressed and sedentary, then becoming overweight. When I test their memories, their scores may fall into the dementia range."

She created a plan for her new patient to follow. It didn't involve any high-tech interventions or groundbreaking medication. She just recommended self-care, some new habits, and a little help from a physical therapist. "Within a year, he was walking 3 to 4 miles a day, and now, years later, he's very trim, he has zero evidence of cognitive impairment, and he has a high quality of life," Dr. Eckstrom says.

Though death steals your most important possession—your life—the aging process that precedes it can commit more minor crimes against you for decades. A little vandalism as it changes your appearance; some petty theft as it raids your muscle mass and energy; and a whole lot of littering as it leaves behind chronic ailments.

You can't outwit death. But you *can* outsmart aging to a degree that too many people overlook.

Living well in the face of aging and illness throughout your forties, fifties, sixties, and beyond requires some of the insight from the previous chapter. You need to find the will to prevent the changes you can control, the ability to adapt to the changes you can't control, and the wisdom to know the difference between the two. Here's how.

Make Any Long-Overdue Adjustments to Your Health Habits

"I recommend a cradle-to-grave approach to healthy living," Dr. Eckstrom says. If you practiced just a small handful of healthy habits "from the day you're born to the day you die, you'd have less chance of having those years of chronic disability and chronic medical conditions."

I'm fairly certain you're familiar with those healthy habits. In fact, I'm hesitant to repeat them here, lest you fall asleep or skip ahead. They're common knowledge. They're clichéd. But it's quite likely that you *haven't* been doing them your whole life.

A 2013 study of US Baby Boomers revealed that they "have higher rates of chronic disease, more disability, and lower self-rated health than members of the previous generation at the same age."[2] Compared to their parents, they were more likely to be obese and less likely to exercise regularly. They were also more likely to walk with a cane and have some sort of disability. But they did smoke less, which is a major plus.

A study the next year found that Boomers also ate more calories, fat, sodium, and cholesterol—in short, "chronic disease–related nutrients"—than the previous generation.[3]

But even if you've been less than careful with your health, you can still make changes that will help you live the coming years and decades on *your* terms, instead of at the mercy of illness and loss of abilities. It's not too late.

Experts call this idea *compression of morbidity.* It means delaying the illnesses and injuries (in other words, morbidity) that reduce your quality of life. If you can push their onset further into the future toward the end of your life, they'll affect you for a briefer period.[4]

In one study that started monitoring seniors starting at age 68 and continued for roughly 20 years, those in the low-risk category (they exercised, didn't smoke, and weren't obese) had markedly less disability during this period than those who were high risk.[5]

In a more recent study, researchers tracked 5,100 British men and women, starting at ages 42 to 63, to see who achieved "successful aging." This meant being mentally sharp and emotionally healthy; free of cancer, heart disease, stroke, and diabetes; and with good lung health and no physical difficulties that impaired their daily activities.[6]

People who practiced four healthy behaviors were more than *three times* more likely to age successfully than people who did none. Those behaviors were being a lifelong nonsmoker, drinking moderately at most, exercising regularly, and eating fruits and vegetables every day.

The more of these habits the participants followed, the more benefit they saw for their bodies and minds. "Our results should motivate lifestyle changes that not only reduce mortality and morbidity, but also improve quality of life at older ages," the researchers wrote.

So . . . are you? Motivated, that is?

If you could make the adjustments to your habits, practices, and body measurements that might boost the quality of this meaningful, happy life you're planning, would you be willing to do so?

Dr. Eckstrom recommends a core set of five health-related behaviors to her patients. If you can immediately switch them all on and keep them going, that's terrific. If you can't, then try setting small, easily attainable goals to help you gradually ramp up these health settings until they're running steadily from day to day.

Follow the Mediterranean diet. This means mostly eating plant-based foods, like fruits and vegetables, whole grains, beans, and nuts. Add some fish, olive oil, and small amounts of cheese and yogurt, and go very light on red meat. That's it.[7]

This diet may have antiaging benefits that go all the way down to your DNA. In 2014, a study involving more than 4,600 healthy female nurses, with an average age of 59, found that those who followed a more Mediterranean-style diet had longer *telomeres*.[8] These are little caps on the chromosomes in your DNA. Telomeres are frequently compared to the plastic nubbins at the ends of shoelaces—which in turn are called *aglets,* for you word nerds—and they serve as markers of how well you're aging. Telomeres naturally grow shorter as you get older, though not everyone's telomeres dwindle at the same rate. Shorter telomeres are linked to a lower life expectancy and a higher risk of age-related disease.

You can't measure the length of your telomeres on your own, but keeping this image in mind can serve as a helpful reminder that the foods you eat *do* make a meaningful difference in your body, even if you can't see it happening.

Keep your body weight close to its ideal. The body mass index (or BMI) isn't a perfect measurement, but it does give you a sense of whether your body weight is in the ideal range. If you know your height and weight, you can easily use a BMI calculator found online to determine yours.

A 2015 review of earlier research found that being overweight more than doubles your risk of osteoarthritis in your knees. Being obese *quadruples* your risk. Knee osteoarthritis can keep you from walking or climbing stairs comfortably, which could eventually lead to a sedentary lifestyle that increases your risk of chronic disease even further, according to the Arthritis Foundation.[9, 10]

Are you carrying too much weight? Just set a goal of losing 5 pounds for now, Dr. Eckstrom suggests. Then apply the habits you're developing and the weight-loss insight you're gathering toward the next 5 pounds, and so forth.

Exercise an hour on most days. This may sound like quite a bit of exercise, but it's probably trifling in comparison to the amount of time you spend sitting down.

Gym Trips Help Senior Stay Vigilant against Long List of Ailments

When Bob Dickerson walks through the gym near his Indianapolis home, people pause what they're doing to watch him. The man simply doesn't seem like the usual 71-year-old.

His hair is snowy, and he has noticeable dings from his encounters with serious illness. Yet the certainty of his stride and the width of his shoulders bring to mind the young Marine and competitive power lifter he once was.

Though Dickerson says he's always enjoyed hard workouts, one of the factors that currently sends him to the gym surprised me. "It's fear. Fear of not being able to combat anything that returns," he says.

In his late fifties, as he was facing quintuple-bypass heart surgery, he promised his wife he'd bounce back. "The fifth day after I came home, Jane told me, 'Tomorrow we're going to walk to the corner.' Sure as shit, we did. Every day we added on, and 6 weeks after my heart surgery, I went back to work. That week I worked 40 hours, plus 30 overtime."

Incidentally, he could still bench-press 300 pounds.

Then he developed cancer in the base of his tongue. During the 3 months he went without solid food while receiving chemotherapy and radiation, he lost 53 pounds. The cancer and its treatments also caused permanent swallowing and speech issues. Shortly before the doctor removed his feeding tube, Dickerson taught himself how to drink a shot of milk and eat a raspberry, with great effort. "It was a celebration," he says. "Jane cried, she was so happy."

Three years later, cancer struck his jaw, requiring an 11-hour surgery to remove the tumor and repair the damage with bone from his lower left leg. But just last year (without Jane's permission) he got on the bench to see how much he could still press. It was 225.

The last time I saw Dickerson at the gym, he was still persevering after the first of two knee replacements, and bystanders were still tracking him. On the phone, he told me he's still trying to stay stronger than whatever crosses his path next.

"Someday that may be more than I can do. But for right now, I can."

Dr. Eckstrom's suggestion corresponds with the recommendations that the American College of Sports Medicine and the American Heart Association published for older adults. They recommend 2½ to 5 hours of aerobic physical activity each week, plus at least two strength-training and flexibility-improving sessions weekly.[11] (Dr. Eckstrom suggests including some tai chi, especially as you get older, because it can reduce your risk of falls, which are a major cause of injury and disability in seniors.)

If you can't exercise that much due to chronic illness or injuries, then get as much physical activity as you can and gradually try to work up to more. Talk to your doctor before beginning to find a plan that's right for you. And try to view exercise as a meaningful use of your time that corresponds to your important values (such as "I want to stay vigorous and active so I can squeeze as much out of this life as I can").

Don't smoke. This one's pretty simple. If you need help quitting, a good way to start is by having a chat with your doctor.

If you drink, keep it moderate. Again, this one is straightforward. Moderate means no more than one drink daily for women or two for men. According to the World Health Organization, more than 5 percent of the world's burden of disease and injury is due to alcohol. If you need help cutting back on drinking, your doctor should be able to assist here, too.[12]

Play an Active Role in Your Healthcare

Here's a fact about healthcare that not everybody knows: For certain medical problems, the solution is obvious. For example, if you break a hip, it needs to be fixed. "For most medical decisions, however, more than one reasonable path forward exists (including the option of doing nothing, when appropriate)," wrote Boston physician Michael Barry, MD, and a colleague in the *New England Journal of Medicine.* Dr. Barry is an expert in an approach called shared decision making.[13]

For those healthcare choices without a clear "right answer," many doctors now recommend that we bring an understanding of our preferences and values to the table so we can contribute to the decision-making process.

For example, let's say rather than breaking your hip, you develop osteo-arthritis in it. Walking becomes painful. One option might be to take an anti-inflammatory drug; another might be a hip replacement. If you're sharing in the decision making, your conversation with the doctor might touch on a variety of factors.[14]

- What activities would you like to resume doing because they bring you happiness or meaning? Are you hoping to do more downhill skiing? Or do you simply want to get back out in your garden? Would one of the treatment options more likely to be a good choice for your needs?

- What are the possible risks that you'll experience complications or that the treatment will fail?

- How much will the treatment cost?

- How much work the options will require (like taking medications daily or going through rehabilitation after a surgery). Are you willing to make this effort? Will you have support through the process, such as from family members?

- The possibility of doing *no* treatment. Perhaps you might just keep an eye on the situation for a while. For example, recent years have seen a steep rise in "watchful waiting"—also called *active surveillance*—in men with prostate cancer that appears to be slow-growing and less threatening. This approach comes with trade-offs, but it can help certain men avoid or delay treatments that can cause unpleasant side effects like incontinence and impotence.[15]

If you haven't been playing an active role in your medical decisions, now is a good time to start practicing. Later on, if you're nearing the end of a terminal illness or you fall critically ill, you or someone speaking on your behalf might need to participate in decisions about life-sustaining treatments. (We'll come back to this in Part Four.) If you've had practice weighing your values, wishes, and goals when making healthcare choices, you and your family may feel more confidence and less distress when facing end-of-life decisions.

Take a Look at Your Medicine Cabinet

One way you can play an important role in your healthcare today is to visit your physician to review your medications. Nearly half of Americans use a prescription medication; 21 percent take three or more; and 10 percent take at least *five*. As you go through your middle and senior years, your odds of using a medication (or several) soar.[16]

These drugs can help you—but they can also cause harm. "The burden of pills is *enormous* in our society, and many of them have side effects that impair your quality of life," Dr. Eckstrom says. Narcotic pain relievers often cause constipation. Many drugs cause nausea, insomnia, or dizziness. Some may cause you to have difficulty thinking clearly. You may end up wanting a treatment for the problems your "helpful" medications cause.

Your doctor may be able to simplify your pill regimen. Or (here's another often-overlooked fact for you), lifestyle changes may help reduce your need for medications for some chronic conditions.

"When I look at someone who's taking 15 pills and they have these problems, I say, 'Let's work together to change your lifestyle and get off some of the medications you're on.' They may be able to get off sleeping pills and narcotic pain pills, and maybe ratchet back their blood pressure pills because they're more active. That makes an enormous difference," Dr. Ekstrom says.

Of course, always do this work with your healthcare provider, rather than experimenting with your medications on your own.

Roll with the Punches

The classic medical handbook *The Merck Manual* cheerfully notes that "most bodily functions peak shortly before age 30 and then begin a gradual but continuous decline." The clear lenses in your eyes stiffen, as do the ligaments in your joints. Accordingly, your vision blurs and your limbs lose flexibility. Your skin grows thinner (hello, wrinkles), your bladder holds less (more overnight restroom visits), and your brain shrinks (thus processing information differently).[17]

More than 20 percent of Americans in the 45-to-64 age group have at least two common chronic conditions, such as high blood pressure, heart disease, diabetes, cancer, or chronic lung disease. After age 65, nearly half of Americans have two or more of these problems.

A healthy lifestyle helps to limit the impact of our bodies' natural physical decline during our later years. But eventually, some age-related changes or chronic ailments are going to get through your defenses. How you respond will be a major determinant in how well you continue to live.[18]

During her academic career, Kathryn Betts Adams, PhD, MSW, has studied how seniors cope, or in some cases don't cope, with age-related health changes. When we spoke, she'd recently left her social work faculty position at Case Western Reserve University in Cleveland.[19]

One response to these changes is to grieve them, she says. "Things happen as you age. You get the wrinkles, the gray hairs, and a lot of people get some type of health problem even by the time they're in their forties," she says. "These changes become harder to accept if we don't allow ourselves to process the grief." (You'll learn more about approaches to grieving in Chapter 9.)

Having a flexible attitude can also help you cope with age-related changes, she says. Some recent research backs this up. In a 2016 study, researchers interviewed 80 people, average age 54, who were living with chronic pain. Based on the patients' stories, the researchers divided them into two groups: Those who displayed a sense of wisdom in their attitude, and those who didn't.[20]

The wisdom group tended to express gratitude for the days they didn't feel pain and for the opportunities to learn and grow from their challenges. Though they often used medication for their pain, they also turned to mind-body practices like yoga, meditation, and pleasurable activities like art, listening to music, and spending time in nature.

"Figuring out how we are out of balance can provide us with clues that will help us heal and/or cope," a 42-year-old said. Of particular interest to this book's conversation, another 40-something participant told the researchers, "I really have gotten in touch with the fragility of life, that physically we're subject to decay and pain. Maybe my fear of death has lessened a little bit because I've gotten in touch with [the fact] that I'm not invulnerable."

The other group tended to discuss more negative emotions, like anger, pessimism, and an inability to forgive. Often they had trouble accepting their situation, relaxing their tension, or finding calm.

In a blog, Dr. Adams wrote that "midlife is a time to reevaluate our health

---

Age-Related Changes That Seem Like a Downer Could Be Signs That You'll Rise

When you're in your older years, you may become less concerned with your body's age-related changes because your focus is on a more meaningful level of your existence.

A theory called *gerotranscendence*—which essentially means "rising above in old age"—holds that some seniors' points of view become elevated above the old habits and attitudes that once defined them and held them in place.[21]

During interviews with older adults, the developer of this idea, a Swedish sociologist named Lars Tornstam, PhD, discovered some recurring themes.

- Elders learn to care for their bodies "without being obsessed" with them. In particular, women spoke of how their earlier focus on beauty gave way to acceptance and more satisfaction with their appearance.
- Elders are less self-centered. In a Swedish survey, 73 percent of older adults said, "Today I take myself less seriously than earlier." The recognition that you're *not* as important as you once thought might someday come as a relief.
- Elders have a better understanding of who they truly are, rather than the roles they've played in their lives. Sometimes seniors are willing to abandon these old roles in order to live more in line with their authentic selves.

So if age spots, sore knees, and gravity are pulling you away from who you once thought you were, perhaps time is carrying you closer to who you truly are.

---

practices, to try to do what we can to feel good and stave off frailty and disability in later life . . . and we hope our lives will be meaningful and that we will have purpose. Midlife is a time to think about our strengths and talents and how we can make the best use of both to please ourselves and serve others."[22]

Whatever your age, if illness or physical decline intrudes on your important activities, find a way to pivot so that you can acknowledge that change and discover new sources of meaning and happiness.

"If we hang on to ideas about how we should be because that's how we were when we were younger, we're going to be stagnated, or bitter, or sad. We need to keep working through that mind-set," Dr. Adams says. "There are tons of examples where people can't do what they used to do, but they do it in some different way." For example, the football player retires and becomes a coach or the concert pianist becomes a teacher.

Let's say a health problem disrupts your routine, as in the pro cyclist's story on page 98—perhaps a chronic injury turns long-distance bicycling from a passion to a source of discomfort. A change in equipment might solve the problem, such as switching to a recumbent bicycle that lets you sit lower on a more padded seat. Or maybe you can find meaning from cycling by helping *other* people enjoy it, such as by volunteering at races in your community or repairing donated bikes for needy kids. Also, analyze the precise reasons why you enjoyed an activity you can't do anymore. Let's say skydiving was a big source of your meaning and happiness. Did it appeal to one of your strengths, such as your self-reliance, your calm, or your attention to detail when repacking your parachute? What other hobbies could utilize these strengths?

Adapting to changes due to illness and aging requires making adjustments that are similar to the questions you asked to find your life's meaning (Chapter 3) or to make your job more of a calling (page 59). What values support your identity and fuel the activities you enjoy? How can you act on these values in new ways? What are new strategies you can roll out to help you support your mission statement? Can you ask someone who's faced a similar life shift to provide some advice and guidance?

Your story is continuing, and I guarantee you've never read a good novel in which the author runs out of ideas and just fills out the remainder of the book with blank pages. Keep writing your story. As long as you're alive, there's *some* activity out there that will bring you happiness and meaning.

As Dr. Adams wrote, "It is through synching the body with the mind through real experience: exercise, sexual intimacy, dance, art- or music-making, cooking real food, playing with children or pets, being outside in nature—anything "analog"—that we keep in touch with our range of emotions, our physical bodies, and our status as humans, a good start toward wisdom at any age."[23]

LIVE WELL, DIE HAPPY EXERCISES
Chapter 6

Now you'll adjust your identity and activities to accommodate changes due to aging, illness, or injury. Copy this section so you can revisit it over time to continually adjust as needed.

Physical Health Settings

I visit my healthcare provider for checkups on a schedule that's ideal for my age and health.

I'm keeping an appropriate visit schedule   **I never visit my healthcare provider**

On a scale of 1 to 10, how well does my diet resemble the Mediterranean diet on page 105?

1	2	3	4	5	6	7	8	9	10

How close am I to a healthy weight?

Markedly below   **Ideal**   **Markedly above**

How much exercise do I get per week?

At least the recommended amount   **None**

Do I smoke?

No   **Occasionally**   **Regularly**

Do I drink?

No   **Moderately**   **Excessively**

How much of a role do I play in my healthcare decisions?

I participate fully in my healthcare decisions   **My doctor makes all or most of my healthcare decisions**

Attitudes and Activities Settings

APPEARANCE

When I think about when I was at my peak attractiveness, what did I particularly like about my appearance? _____

_____

_____

_____

What behaviors, activities, or attitudes did my appearance support (like flirting, dating, carrying myself with confidence)? _____

_____

_____

_____

Compared to then, how has my appearance changed? _____

_____

_____

_____

Are these earlier behaviors, activities, or attitudes still important for me to maintain?

_____

_____

_____

If yes, what other qualities do I have—or could I develop—that would help me continue these behaviors, activities, or attitudes? _____

_____

_____

_____

If no, what new behaviors, activities, or attitudes could I develop that would provide happiness and meaning, given my appearance today? _____

_____

_____

_____

PHYSICAL ACTIVITIES

When I think about when I had my peak physical abilities, what physical activities did I particularly enjoy doing? _____

_____

_____

_____

Compared to then, how have my physical abilities changed? _____

_____

_____

_____

Are those earlier physical activities still important for me to do? _____

_____

_____

_____

If yes, how can I continue to participate in those activities—or find related activities that provide a similar sense of meaning and happiness—given my current physical abilities?_____

_____

_____

_____

If no, what other uses of my time would provide me happiness and meaning, given my physical abilities today? _____

_____

_____

_____

_____

Part 3

A BRIEF DETOUR TO YOUR EVENTUAL DEPARTURE

It's time to start shifting the focus from living well to dying happy. But even though you flipped a page to start this section, you're not completely switching topics. Life and death remain entwined and inseparable.

In this section, you'll glance forward to your potential Point B—literally, the end of your line—so you can chart the clearest, best path to get you to where you'd like to be at the end.

In Chapter 7, you'll learn how to tap into the experiences of people who are nearer the endpoint—people who are quite old, or dying, or both—to help you plot your course. They're like online reviewers who have visited the tourist hotspots you're considering. If you see enough complaints, that's a good reason to steer away from one particular destination. Conversely, if you see enough positive reviews from people who seem knowledgeable, it's worth considering whether you'd like to go there, too.

In Chapter 8, you'll start planning what you want to leave behind: the memories, values, mementos, and resources that create your legacy. After you're gone, this version of you can continue—serving as a testament to the time you were alive, and providing comfort to the people you loved.

CHAPTER 7

Dodge the Common Sources of Deathbed Distress

The elderly woman dying in the hospice was born before the Titanic sank and not so long after the Wright brothers' first flight. She witnessed the advent of radio, the Internet, the interstate highway system, and space travel. She outlasted nearly everyone who was alive when she was born, and over the course of her 100-plus years, the planet's population quadrupled.

Yet at the end, she told the hospice chaplain, Kerry Egan, that she was amazed it was nearly over. "She even laughed when she said it: 'Somehow I thought I'd have more time!'" Egan told me.[1]

Egan, who shared the lessons she's learned from listening to people at the end of life in her book *On Living,* says she frequently hears this sentiment. "Everyone seems to think they were going to have more time. It's this expression of incredible surprise."

The end of life also finds some people struggling with unresolved guilt and regret. Sometimes we use these words interchangeably, but they're technically two different flavors of distress. Guilt, by one definition from the *American Journal of Hospice & Palliative Medicine,* occurs when "healthy persons violate their consciences." It's the feeling that you've done wrong, that you've acted counter to your values and principles. "Regret, on the other hand, is the feeling of sadness that accompanies choices that do not turn out as intended."[2]

Even though our time becomes short at the end, we may have more opportunity to replay our life's choices if we're lying in bed or in a recliner and we're no longer occupied with our daily tasks.

Though some common themes tend to emerge at the end of life (as you'll see in the sidebar on page 128), the sources of regret and guilt you may someday feel will be unique to *you*. Will you wish you'd spent your time differently? That you had explored more? That you had seen the world more clearly?

Amy Getter, MS, RN, a hospice nurse in Oregon, watches many people work through this type of self-examination before they die.[3]

"I'd say the biggest regrets that people have discussed with me are situations with loved ones that didn't go well, people they wish they'd stayed in contact with, and estrangement from family members. Sometimes they feel like they wasted a lot of time."

One man in his late fifties with whom she had worked, who died over the holidays, had struggled with alcoholism for years. "When he got his terminal diagnosis, he finally stopped drinking. His take on it was, 'Why didn't I do this sooner? Why didn't I realize what an impact my drinking had on my family?'

"But what the family said was that 'We got these 5 months! We had these amazing conversations.' It was amazing that this man in his last weeks and months was able to come to terms with all this regret, and yet take away something sweet and give to his family. Lots of people have that experience," she says.

Remember: Even when you're dying, you're still alive. Even if you're sick and struggling, you can accomplish great things in a short amount of time.

But—and this is an important *but*—you may not get this chance to address your sources of regret or guilt at the end of your life. You could die suddenly. Dementia could undermine the clarity of your thoughts long before your final breath. Or the physical and emotional challenges of dying could preoccupy your mind.

So why not work through any regret or guilt now? Why not set yourself up so that if you have some space at the end, it's available for honoring and celebrating the things that went right?

"I've had lots of patients over the years who shared with me the things they were really happy they were able to do, like travel to other places or have jobs like teaching and a feeling like they had given back to their students over the years. Some were medical people who felt they'd made a difference, or parents who were proud of what their kids had done," Getter says.

"I think there are all these aspects of accomplishing the things we care about, and oftentimes at the end people show it with their grandkids' pictures or a photo of their daughter winning a spelling bee," she says.

If you take a proactive approach to your guilt and regret today, the benefits don't just come at this future point—they can start immediately.

"People can have a million regrets at the end, which means you can be *free* from a million regrets now!" Egan says, her voice rising with excitement. "If you regret that you never told your mother that you forgive her for X, Y, or Z, how sad it would be to have to live with that regret! If there are things you want to do, do them! If there are relationships you want to repair, do it now. Then you get to enjoy the fruits of that effort!"

Also, remember the advice from the retired pastor and widower in the introduction of this book: If you want to learn how to die well, you have to practice learning to live with loss. Your losses will occur with regularity over your life, and it's important to find a way to fit them into your life story as you go.

"No one gets to decide what losses they will face. Nobody chooses to lose a child. Nobody chooses to have a terrible neurodegenerative disease," Egan says. "But you do get to choose what it means. That's the work of meaning-making. That's why you should do it now. If people feel like the suffering in their life had no meaning, that's painful."

It's likely that you'll reach your deathbed with *some* sort of second-guessing. But by following the four strategies in this chapter, you'll improve your chances of reaching the end with fewer painful burdens to occupy the dwindling time that you could devote elsewhere.

The first strategy is to find teachers who are near the end themselves. Fortunately, they're not hard to track down.

Guilt and Regret Reliever #1:
Find a Mentor Who Knows about
Aging and Dying

Long ago, Kim Mooney had a brush with cancer. "I started to go through an intense grief process. I hadn't thought about dying before, and all of a sudden I'm facing my own death. Well, I wasn't *close* to death, but everyone in my cancer support group died but me," she says. "I decided I needed to get more information about what was going on before it was right in my face."[4]

Mooney wanted to take the mystery out of death, so when it did arrive, she'd be prepared. So she started volunteering at a hospice. She ended up facilitating bereavement and education services in Boulder, Colorado, and now she does similar work through her own business, Practically Dying.

She urges people to start contemplating death—their own and others'—while they're still well "upstream" from the end of their life. A good way to do so is to spend time regularly around the elderly and the dying.

"I think when we're around older people and we're paying attention, we get the wisdom of their life. I sit with people in their eighties. They've seen their friends die, and they've come to accept that it's normal, and that's how we start to make peace with death," she says.

While visiting long-term care facilities in the days after September 11, 2001, she found that the TVs were tuned to the video footage of jets making impact and buildings falling, over and over.

"I was sitting next to this older woman, and at one point, she reached out and put her hand on mine and said, 'Don't worry, we're going to get through this.' It was so comforting to me. She didn't tell me this part, but she was a Holocaust survivor. The breadth and depth of her experience just showed up," she says.

Marc Agronin, MD, a geriatric psychiatrist, director of mental health and clinical research at a long-term care facility in Miami, and author of *How We Age: A Doctor's Journey into the Heart of Growing Old,* also found his way into his profession by first spending time in a nursing home.[5]

"When I was in high school, I volunteered in a nursing home. I got to know this older man in his eighties. I was so moved by him that he shaped my life," he says. "There's nothing he told me or did that was earth-shattering. For me, being around older people is similar to how people talk about being in nature. There's just this sense you have of what life is about."

You can find these sorts of teachers in hospice care facilities. Roughly 1.6 million people at the end of life received hospice services in 2014, and the number keeps growing. Hospice organizations are required by Medicare rules to recruit volunteers for administrative or patient-facing roles.[6, 7]

As a volunteer, you don't have to do any hands-on healthcare or personal care tasks. Hospice clients simply need you to *be* there, according to the Hospice Foundation of America. You might read to patients, listen to their stories, visit with their families, or sing to them alone or with a chorus of friends.[8]

Be the One Who Keeps Someone from Dying Alone

Yet another way to provide comfort to someone at the end of life, and develop a deeper understanding of the process for yourself, is to volunteer for No One Dies Alone. This is a national program that many hospitals offer.[9]

The program is designed to provide companionship for patients who are actively dying but don't have loved ones available to be with them in their final days. (This can happen for a variety of reasons: They've outlived their spouse; their family is traveling from a distance; they fell ill away from home; or their loved ones are too distraught to be present.)

Again, you don't provide medical or nursing care; you simply make a commitment to be there for a few hours to hold the patient's hand, pray if appropriate, listen if they're talking, and bear witness to the end of their life.

You may find that the time you spend around people at the end of life is personally enriching. One recent study, which reviewed earlier research, showed that hospice volunteering can help you find "a greater appreciation of what is really important in life."[10] Research also shows that spending time in a hospice environment can help you grow more comfortable with your own mortality. In a study of 23 volunteers, some said they had grown more accepting of the idea of dying.[11]

Another 1.4 million people were in nursing homes in 2014, which also typically welcome volunteers who can come in to play music, bring well-behaved and approved pets to snuggle with residents, or visit residents.[12] Or you can spend time visiting with an older person who is still living at home. A number of Web sites—including Create the Good and Elder Helpers—can put you in touch with senior associations that are looking for volunteers in your area.

By spending time with seniors, you can:

- Provide a valuable service to people who need assistance and companionship

- Discuss the choices they made that enhanced their life's meaning—as well as decisions that have led to guilt and regret

- Give them another way to stay connected with the world. We all want to feel like we have a purpose for being alive, even when our ability to work or care for others is diminished. When you show up, you may give someone a chance to feel valuable by sharing their wisdom or providing a firsthand account of a bygone era with few remaining eyewitnesses.

Guilt and Regret Reliever #2: Work on Your Current Sources of Distress

Years ago, doctors, mental healthcare providers, and social workers noticed a curious development. Aging veterans who were facing big changes in their senior years, such as retirement or terminal illness, were struggling with more anguish over their wartime experiences.[13]

Though some veterans had shown symptoms of post-traumatic stress disorder (PTSD) following their service, many had not suffered from it during the previous decades of civilian life. Some researchers gave this resurfacing distress the name *late-onset stress symptomatology,* or LOSS.

Bothered by the Idea of Being Old?
Try This Approach

"I'm grateful for every moment I have," a gray-haired senior told George Costanza over a bowl of soup in a classic *Seinfeld* episode. A baffled George sputtered in outrage, "How can you be so grateful when you're so close to the end?"[14]

In real life, some research has found that seniors tend to have less anxiety about death. If you want to find out why, you might learn by volunteering with them. (But try to be more tactful than Costanza was.)

Another fan of looking to older people as mentors for living well and dying happy is Nick Carleton, PhD, the "intolerance of uncertainty" expert you met earlier. "Go talk to seniors. They've got a way better perspective on it," he says. "They're not sitting there gripping the armchair with worry, at least the ones I've had the pleasure of interacting with."[15]

Part of the reason could be that many seniors have learned to tolerate more uncertainty as they get older, he says. When changes arise that are out of their control, they have more practice handling them.

Plus over the decades, they may have found other reasons to welcome their mortality: Perhaps they're envisioning relief from pain, or a chance to reunite with departed loved ones. Ask them!

If the present version of yourself who's young and healthy (or at least young*ish* and healthy*ish*) has trouble coping with the idea of someday being near the end of life, now is a good time to start working on it. Finding wise elders is a reasonable place to begin.

This sort of discomfort over events from long ago may arise late in life because that's when people in general, not just veterans, tend to do more "life review." In this process, you sort through memories to see how they fit into your life's meaning or purpose. This may involve looking through yearbooks and photo albums, visiting important sites from your life, or telling stories to your grandkids. "Maybe I have more time on my hands or maybe as we get older—when we're young and we're 40 or 50, [we]'re not thinking of older years or death or illness," one WWII veteran told a researcher. Another noted, "As we now reach a certain point in our lives, certain things come to mind ... We seem to reflect more."

Another reason why events from the past may become especially painful later in life, according to researchers, is because the deaths of loved ones or the loss of your vigor or health may bring up memories of painful losses from earlier in your life.

Death Announcements Offer Useful Life Guidance

If you want to find the more common sources of regret and guilt that people have at the end of life, reading a few obituaries can be highly enlightening. Here are some causes of distress collected from the nation's obits on Legacy.com over a recent 1-year period.[16]

- Never going on safari or visiting Australia.
- Leaving the police department.
- Being an absent father and husband.
- Not using an inheritance to go to college.
- "My two divorces and the families that were broken."
- "Regrets, I've had a few; but then again, too few to mention."
- "That he never found the time to see the Chairman (Frank Sinatra) in person."
- "Most who knew me thought me fairly talented, but the consensus of those same people was that I was by no stretch of the imagination nice. They were right, and I died—Thursday, at age 67, by the way—with more than my share of regret."
- "When his children were born, he was so in love with each of them but lost touch through the years, something he regretted and was hoping to change."
- That the Spanish Civil War prevented his pursuit of advanced classical guitar studies.

"Often, my job is to work with people who feel that way. They feel a deep sense of regret, or anger, or fury sometimes at their current circumstances, and sometimes at disappointments in life or tragedies they've faced," Dr. Agronin says. These residents include veterans who've seen brutal combat, survivors of the Holocaust, and immigrants who left their personal connections and worldly possessions behind when they fled.

"Sometimes when late life is rough, it's not something new. It's a process

- "To his children, Bud's biggest regret was not spending enough time with and truly getting to know each of you; he sincerely hoped for forgiveness from you; you were loved and in years to come his hope was that you would know that."
- Being unable to continue his education because he needed to work to support his family in the midst of the Great Depression.
- "Picking up a cigarette, because of the amount of time it stole from her happiness."
- Missing the opportunity to take piano lessons.
- Not learning how to swim.
- Never learning to drive a car.
- Being unable to take her great-grandchild to Disney due to her brain cancer.
- "That I was so busy when you kids were small that I barely remember that time. I worked so hard, and time just got by me. I don't remember talking to you or listening, really. If I could do it over again, I'd slow down and enjoy those years when you were children . . . I feel like I still don't know how to talk to you, and I feel like I've missed half of your lives."
- "Not having more time with his children, and not being able to make things right."

that's been going on for years, if not decades. Someone may have depression that's recurred, or they have substance abuse issues," he says. "Most of these individuals, if you turn the clock back 30 years, you'd see the same issues, and for some reason they didn't get the help they needed at the time or weren't able to resolve it."

Taking a cue from those who face late-in-life guilt or regret, perhaps doing some life review would be useful to you *now.* What stressful events have you been through? What big jolts, losses, or threats to your safety or well-being have you endured? These might be issues that had an obvious effect on your peace of mind at the time, or you may have been able to deal with them well enough that they didn't interfere with your daily life. Also, are you struggling with ongoing grief? Depression? Anxiety? Anger? Substance abuse?

These sources of distress could darken the end of your life, either because they continue unabated or they resurface when a less-busy schedule leaves you with more time to reflect and ruminate.

If you suspect that you have any issues that could benefit from sessions with a counselor, therapist, or support group, don't put off your search for relief. Look for it now.

Guilt and Regret Reliever #3: Deal with Family Estrangement

In many cases, guilt and regret grow in the space between parents and grown children, especially when that space becomes wide.

San Francisco–based psychologist Joshua Coleman, PhD, the author of *When Parents Hurt,* told me that most family estrangements develop for just a handful of reasons.[17]

In 75 percent of the cases he sees, divorce caused the rift, whether it occurred when the offspring were children or adults. One parent in a divorced couple might poison a child's relationship with the other parent. Or a child may form a tighter bond with a parent who seems damaged and fragile, and thus seems to need help. A child who feels that one parent came out of the divorce the "winner" may side with the other parent out of anger or sympathy. Or after the divorce, kids of any age may see their parents more as individuals rather than a family unit of which they're a part.

Another common reason why adult children become estranged is because their spouse demands distance. "Sometimes the parent is critical of a son-in-law or daughter-in-law, and that sets things off on the wrong foot. But also sometimes the kid marries someone who's troubled or controlling; they may basically tie the adult child up in knots psychologically so they feel like they have to choose between the parent and the spouse. That's common," he says.

Mental illness or substance abuse—on either party's end—can cause estrangement. So can natural shifts in the relationship that occur as the child reaches adulthood and seeks independence. "Often it can be that the kid doesn't know any other way to separate from a parent aside from rejecting them," he says.

If you have a gap in your relationship with an adult child, the following steps may help you begin a healing process to close the gaps. (You can modify these strategies to help address estrangement in other close relationships, too.)

Take their complaints seriously. If you get the chance to hear your child's explanation for an estrangement, listen with an open mind, Dr. Coleman urges. This isn't the time to argue your case.

"In general, I think parents need to take their adult children's complaints seriously. Today, the child gets as much of a vote in what kind of childhood they had as the parent does. If your kid wants to talk about mistakes you made when they were growing up—or now as an adult—be empathetic and listen for the kernel of truth," Dr. Coleman says. "Don't just get defensive and try to prove them wrong, or tell them they're not remembering the great things you did as a parent. Try to see it as an effort on their part to be closer to you through talking about the relationship. Their goal typically isn't to tear down the parent, even when it feels like that."

Ask whether you're truly estranged. Often, parents who see new space between themselves and their grown children don't recognize that this may be normal and even healthy, Dr. Coleman says. When they seek more closeness, the parents' efforts may look like criticism, and the adult child may come away with a sense of guilt. Neither sentiment will add warmth to the relationship.

Remember that your adult child has his own life, and that his studies, marriage, work responsibilities, child-rearing, or other demands are important priorities. Let your kids know that you're interested in adapting the relationship to meet everyone's evolving needs, and ask them what this arrangement would look like to them.

Address the spouse directly. If your child's spouse or romantic partner seems to be the source of the estrangement, offer a conciliatory message to this person. "If your son-in-law or daughter-in-law is sabotaging the relationship, they're the gatekeeper. You can't go around them—you have to go through them!" he laughs.

You could send a letter to just your daughter- or son-in-law, or write to both the spouse and your child. (Or write an e-mail that goes to both, so everyone knows what the others are reading.) "Tell them, 'I assume there are things I've done that are hurtful. I want you to know that I'm interested in what you think and feel. I promise to listen to it in a spirit of understanding you better and making my communication better,'" Dr. Coleman says. "Just basically make it safe for them to complain about you."

This approach may get the relationship moving in a happier direction. And "sometimes if the daughter- or son-in-law is really dedicated to ruining the relationship, it can strengthen the spine of your kid if you show you're willing to do the hard work."

Pause before you change your will. It's not uncommon for parents to want to cut estranged children out of their wills. Dr. Coleman says he typically urges clients not to make this revision. Again, you could be overlooking *your* role in the estrangement. Or your child could genuinely want a better relationship but be unable to say so due to a spouse's involvement or some other factor not fully in her control—and changing the terms of your will would punish your child forever.

This move would also affect your legacy. Altering your will is a final statement that can solidify the way your child—and perhaps grandchildren, too—remembers you forever. "I think one is sending a much stronger message of legacy by leaving a child in the will," he says. You might say, "I'm sad we couldn't connect when I was alive, but I know you wouldn't have done this without a good reason from your perspective. I only wish you a long, healthy life."

Finally, cutting a child out of your will could prevent her from reconciling with her siblings or other family members; it's a loud announcement that "you're not part of this family" that you can never take back. Plus, your estranged child might file legal action against your estate that would put an added burden on your grieving family.

Move on. Remember that your life isn't all about your kids. Give this estrangement the attention it deserves, but try to keep it from entirely filling your field of vision, Dr. Coleman urges.

"Try to make sure it doesn't become a blight on your life. People take their job as parents seriously. If they feel that their child doesn't love them, they may stop having a joyful and meaningful life. No matter what's happening, you can take charge of it to the extent that you're able to compartmentalize it. Most parents, mothers especially, feel like they have to think about their kids all the time if it's not going well, and that's not necessarily a good idea."

Set the stage for resolution as well as you can; in the meantime, redirect your energies to the other areas in your life that provide meaning.

Guilt and Regret Reliever #4: Return to Your Personal Settings Exercises

All the elements on your Personal Settings exercises at the ends of Chapters 4, 5, and 6 are there for a reason. By adjusting how you spend your time; regularly directing your attention to forgiveness, mindfulness, acceptance, and tolerance of uncertainty; and living fully in the face of aging and illness, you're naturally going to accumulate less regret and guilt along the way.

That's because you're living deliberately and paying attention to the important elements in your life. You're pursuing meaning and happiness. You're not adrift, operating on autopilot, and overlooking the opportunities to say or do the right thing.

So revisit those chapters regularly. Do you want to develop a new skill? Do you need to set new goals? Do you need to address a fear that's holding you back or a grudge that's weighing you down?

Do it *now*. Later may be too late.

LIVE WELL, DIE HAPPY EXERCISES
Chapter 7

1. Consider devoting some of your volunteer time to helping people who are elderly or dying. You might see someone getting through a difficult phase in life gracefully—and these lessons could be useful to you if you're ever in a similar situation.

2. Is an old trauma still causing you pain, or can you see how one could reemerge someday if you have more time alone with your thoughts? Have any of your words or actions caused you lingering embarrassment or guilt? Find a way to start reconciling these issues that works for your situation—perhaps by visiting a mental health professional or asking forgiveness from (or offering it to) the people involved.

3. Talk to your loved ones about anything *they* feel guilt or regret about that involves you. Perhaps you could help absolve them of feelings that would cause them distress after you're gone.

CHAPTER 8

Bolster Your Legacy

The Library of Congress doesn't just hold books, nor does it only concern itself with the history of America's most powerful residents and prominent events. If you walk into the library's Thomas Jefferson Building in Washington, DC, and enter the American Folklife Center Reading Room on the ground floor, you can sit down and listen to stories of ordinary, everyday, *fascinating* people.[1]

These recorded stories flow into the library from an organization called StoryCorps. Since 2003, it's collected more than 60,000 interviews from individuals. The organization operates several recording booths around the country and offers a smartphone app for do-it-yourself historians.[2]

The organization's mission is "to preserve and share humanity's stories in order to build connections between people and create a more just and compassionate world," while at the same time "creating an invaluable archive for future generations." It asks storytellers to bring someone into the booth with them—like a family member—to ask questions or serve as an audience, creating a conversation that flows between people. (The booth is equipped with tissues, since tears often flow, too.)[3,4]

A wife opens up to her Army veteran husband about how his PTSD affected her. A mom tells her 8-year-old daughter about giving birth to her while serving a stint in the Rikers Island jail. A man with Alzheimer's disease locates a few of his remaining memories to share with his daughters. He's now gone, and the daughters told StoryCorps that they listen to the recording often.[5, 6, 7]

Humans are "storytelling beings," Dena Huisman, PhD, told me. She's an associate professor at the University of Wisconsin–La Crosse who has studied family storytelling (and also, relevant to this book, how people talk about their grief). Our stories help us "make sense of our lives in a series of starting and ending points," she says. They allow us to organize our experiences into categories. Through stories, we process the meaning of the changes that happen to us.[8]

And, "at the end of life, if we're scared of what happens next, the easiest way to manage that uncertainty is to look back and process your life and tell others about it so you'll be present even when you're absent," she says.

When you go online to learn about legacy planning, you'll find a lot of information about splitting your investments among your heirs, reducing estate taxes, setting up trusts, and other property and money issues. Even a major dictionary defines legacy as: "something (such as property or money) that is received from someone who has died."[9]

It is indeed essential to do the financial planning that distributes your possessions to the people and organizations you care about. We'll touch on those issues, but if you're looking for in-depth guidance, that's the subject of a different book, and you can find many of them.

In this chapter, let's talk about legacy planning in the sense of creating what Dr. Huisman described: an echo that you deliberately send out into the world so you'll be present even when you're absent. The strength of your legacy can come from stories, of course, as well as good examples for others to follow, wise advice, and objects that will connect your loved ones to their heritage after they lose the link that you provided.

Retell Stories That Connect Yesterday with Today

Barbara Greenspan Shaiman's family story has an element that even strangers may find fascinating: It's connected to a much larger event that Steven Spielberg depicted in an Oscar-winning movie.[10, 11]

"My father and grandfather worked for Oskar Schindler (played by Liam Neeson in the movie *Schindler's List*) in his factory in Krakow, Poland. They were fortunate to receive shelter and protection from him. When we came to America, he had no money and didn't speak English, and we had to bring in boarders to help pay rent," she says. "Even when he and his friends who also worked for Schindler were making $35 a week, they would take out a few dollars, and once a month my father would collect it and send Schindler money in gratitude for saving them. They showed their values by always being grateful for someone who did something so heroic for them."

When Shaiman told her 8-year-old granddaughter the story about the boarders, the girl thought she meant the bookstore Borders. "She asked me, 'Oh, you liked to read! Did you go to Barnes and Noble, too?'"

So Shaiman explained the concept of sharing living expenses with strangers, which led to the rest of the story.

"I think my granddaughter needs to understand the resiliency that was imbued in me by my family. This strength that we will prevail, we will do well, in spite of what happened to us," she says.

For a 2014 study, Dr. Huisman spent 6 weeks sifting through family interviews in the StoryCorps archives in the Library of Congress. She chose 119 at random, transcribed them, and found five general themes that loved ones communicate to each other via stories.[12]

Our family endured tough times. Most of the stories portrayed relatives helping each other through difficult situations. In one story, an older woman accompanied by her sister told her daughter how they endured their stepfather's abusive name-calling when they were teens.

These stories often contained a self-help element. Older family members showed younger ones how to solve problems. They often used humor, which can help us process frustrating and threatening experiences. "Boy, we should have done all that stuff he [the stepfather] accused us of!" the older sisters told the younger woman.

And they typically ended on a positive note, much like Shaiman's story of her father repaying his rescuer. The final message is: "We got through this."

Our family has strong internal connections. Elders reminisced about the rituals and in-jokes that defined the family and set it separate from the outside world. Frequently, people spoke with fondness about extended relatives, while showing special favor for their nuclear family. The message they told in these stories is, "Our family has a bond that makes us special."

Our family continues across generations. We tend to have a complicated relationship with older relatives, Dr. Huisman says. We may see them as wise and worthy of honor, yet also exasperating and sometimes boring. (For the latter, she points to Grandpa from *The Simpsons,* once featured in a newspaper under the headline, "Old Man Yells at Cloud.")

The StoryCorps interviews frequently held family elders up to a high standard. The tellers often suggested—or mentioned outright—that future generations would someday join this group as valued members. With their stories, " . . . the present family began the process of idealizing the current generations for future family members," Dr. Huisman wrote.

Our family has been influenced by our culture. Stories often told how world events like the Great Depression or World War II had altered the course of the family, perhaps as a way to help the listener understand and accept the group's beliefs and customs.

Elders also discussed their or their ancestors' immigrant experiences or participation in a particular religion. Such stories show that families can celebrate having links to multiple cultural institutions. (Remember from Chapter 1 that belonging to age-old institutions can help reduce your dread of dying.)

Our family works hard. Storytellers spoke of laboring on the family farm or helping run the family business or household. Their parents and grandparents taught them the value of hard work, and now they're taking the opportunity to pass these lessons on to the younger generation.

The message is that "hard work may not be easy or fun, but it is a valued part of life because it teaches skills for dealing with life," Dr. Huisman wrote.

Want to tell stories that are so durable they'll echo around your grandchildren's dining rooms decades from now? Keep these storytelling rules in mind.

Make it quick. Dr. Huisman is a fan of the "power of everyday storytelling," she says, having learned that the opportunities to best connect with loved ones usually "aren't in grand moments. Most come at the dinner table or when you're in the car. Don't make it, 'I'm going to tell 20 stories in a row.' Tell them for 5 to 10 minutes here and there."

Structure it properly. No one likes to hear a rambling joke without a funny payoff, and no one will want to hear a story that goes nowhere. Your anecdote needs an interesting starting point. It must flow in a way that makes sense. It needs some sort of purpose, like a moral that it teaches. And it needs to land on a solid ending—which can be that moral of the story—Dr. Huisman says.

If you're an unsure raconteur, you can find plenty of skilled examples to follow. Listen carefully to how your favorite comedians, authors, and songwriters structure their stories. The podcast world is also giving us a golden age of storytelling. Check out shows like *This American Life, The Moth,* and *Radiolab* on a service such as iTunes or Stitcher for an education on how to tell a tale that grabs the listener.

Keep it relevant. "If grandparents want their grandchildren to remember a story, it had better have a lasting impact on that generation," Dr. Huisman says. You know this yourself. You can happily watch a movie set 800 years ago, as long as it has a romance or other themes that are meaningful to your life, she adds.

Tie your recollections into advice or wisdom your audience can actually use. How did you impress the boss at your first job? How did you handle a breakup? How did you first woo your spouse? (Side note: Don't actually use the word "woo.") How did you cope with the sickness or death of someone you cared about?

Tolerate repetition. Your audience may want to hear a story over and over. Indulge them. Provide some of the details, but let them add their favorite moments, too. This repetition will help reinforce your story in their mental records.

Preserve your words. With just a computer and webcam, or a digital audio recorder, you can easily set up your own studio to capture your story. Bring in a younger relative to interview you for the camera or recorder, and you'll create a memento that can live indefinitely on a hard drive, in the cloud, or on YouTube.

How should you start? On the StoryCorps Web site, you'll find a list of "great questions" that can prompt dozens of stories. If you want to share more insight into your thought processes and sense of right and wrong, I like

Gregory Stock's *The Book of Questions,* which asks you to tell what you'd do in a variety of morally challenging situations.

Remember the Matriarchs, Too

Another theme that professor Dena Huisman, PhD, discovered when listening to families' stories is that the dads and grandpas played starring roles while the moms and grandmas seldom appeared.

Seriously. We can do better than this. As you're rummaging through your mental files, find meaningful stories to share about *all* the people who played a loving role in your life. The next generations need to hear about the moms, grandmas, and aunts who helped build the family they see around them.

Finally, don't forget to *be* the audience while you still can. During class, Dr. Huisman urges her college students to go call their grandparents. Even if you're no longer a young adult, if you still have parents, grandparents, aunts, or uncles, keep collecting their stories.

You may find that later in life they're motivated to share more details with you. Now that you're an adult, you might hear a more candid story that ventures into areas of family history that were off-limits when you were younger. So be ready for what you could find behind a door when a loved one opens it.

Also, remember this: If your older relative is near the end of life or has a terminal illness or severe limitation, your request for a story provides her with a chance to *give* something of value during a time when she may feel like she's doing a lot of *taking* from her caregivers. These conversations at the end can provide people with a continuing sense of meaning and purpose.

Create a Different Kind of Will

Years ago, attorney Jo Kline Cebuhar, JD, learned of a concept called an *ethical will* while volunteering in a hospice.[13]

This is a document that you leave for your heirs or other important people. (It's not a legal document, by the way.) It can have many components, but Cebuhar recommends that it include at least three parts: your beliefs and values; the lessons you've learned to be true from your own experience; and your hopes for the future, either for your loved ones or for your own life. Her book *So Grows the Tree: Creating an Ethical Will* is one of several she's written about end-of-life concerns.

The Jewish tradition of ethical wills dates back to the Bible's book of Genesis. Here, Jacob assembles his 12 sons and tells them what their future holds, based on their qualities that he admires or finds offensive. He then lies down in bed and dies.

Randy Pausch's "last lecture" video is another type of ethical will, Cebuhar says. The year before he died of pancreatic cancer, the college professor gave a stirring presentation that went viral (it now has more than 18 million views on YouTube) and became a best-selling book. He honored mentors by retelling their wisdom; shared stories of adversities he overcame; and left a meaningful time capsule for his three young children to revisit later.[14, 15]

Interested in using this important tool to strengthen your legacy? Here's how.

Consider starting now. You don't have to wait until you're late in life to create your ethical will, Cebuhar says. Some people find that major transitions—a first child, an empty nest, retirement—are a good time to write about where they've been and what lessons they've learned there. You can add updates to your ethical will over time so your loved ones can see how your thinking progressed, or you can start anew periodically.

Review your beliefs and values. The self-reflection needed for this project can be difficult for some people to muster, Cebuhar says. It requires knowing the values that drive you. How have you tried to improve the world? What do you believe in strongly enough to showcase in this document?

But hopefully, this will be easy for you to discern, since you've done it already. Reread your mission statement on pages 52–53. Think about the improvements you'd like to see in society and the strengths you have that could help make them a reality (page 53). Consider the elements of your job that make it feel like a calling (page 59). Replay the stories of how you learned the life lessons you'd like your descendants to know. Think about the ideas they might find most useful.

Jot all of this down in one place, and you'll be well on your way to creating your ethical will.

Add more. Feel free to go beyond the three core elements that Cebuhar recommends. Some people add ingredients like:

- An effort to make amends with individuals by name or to ask forgiveness from them

- An offering of thanks

- An explanation of their *actual* will. You can offer reasons why you divided your estate like you did; tell the story of heirlooms you bequeathed; or offer suggestions for how your heirs could use the money you left to accomplish meaningful goals.

- Lessons they've learned at the end of life. If you're in this position, have you made discoveries about dying well that could help your family? Developed new spiritual insight during this part of your journey? Learned to see death in a less scary light?

- Words that might heal old estrangements or prevent new ones. Want to reach out to a stubbornly distant sibling? If your feelings were sincere enough to put in this document, perhaps they can provide reconciliation later. Afraid your child won't have a good connection with another family member when you're gone? Perhaps you can offer your blessing to their relationship.

Be creative. Your ethical will can take many forms, which is particularly good for people who aren't comfortable writing, Cebuhar says. You can make a video, a photo scrapbook with comments, a pile of handwritten letters, or even a collection of quotes and song lyrics that describe how you feel.

Stay positive. Though Jacob gave three of his sons a tongue-lashing in Genesis, keep negative comments out of your ethical will, Cebuhar advises. These words are going to last a long time, and after you're gone, you won't have a chance to take them back or soften their delivery.

Share it now or later. You can leave your ethical will in a safe or with a loved one to be opened after your death. Or you can share it while you're alive. It's your choice.

Another Reason to Create an Ethical Will

The thought process required to write an ethical will is a good first step to take in your estate and end-of-life planning, attorney Jo Klein Cebuhar, JD, says. The self-awareness you get from this exercise can help you better understand the value-inspired philanthropic benefit your estate could accomplish, and it may give you some insight into how long you might want to fight a terminal illness.

Live Your Legacy Out Loud

Barbara Shaiman, MEd, who leads workshops about leaving one's legacy, is less focused on what lingers after you die and more eager that you ... well, it's the title of her book: *Live Your Legacy Now!*

"People come up to me and say, 'My dad just died, and we were going through his belongings. We didn't know he did *this* and did *that*.' They're angry," she says. "Why did they not know that? Why are people leaving it to their family to put the pieces of the puzzle together and say, 'This is what Mom or Dad or Joe were about'?"

Over the course of our conversation, she mentioned many of the components of a meaningful and happy life that you have encountered in previous chapters. By sharing these details about yourself, you can witness the creation of your legacy as you're living it.

If you hit an obstacle that limits your ability to enjoy your passion, help *other* people appreciate it. Does a bad shoulder hamper your golf swing? A friend of Shaiman's who is an avid golfer teaches blind people to play. Now that your family is scattered, do you miss the chance to cook big meals? She met a woman with a passion for cooking who vowed to teach her 20-something son with Down syndrome and his friends how to cook so they can be more self-sufficient.

When you volunteer in your community, make a donation, or offer a helping hand, include the younger generations in your effort. If you inspire them to follow your lead, their efforts to do good down the road will likely evoke memories of your example.

In short, as you're making discoveries about who you are and who you want to become, celebrate them! You don't have to tell the world about your good deeds in a boastful way. Simply show what you're doing.

"If you're not feeling good about your legacy while you're alive, you can change it. Once you're dead, it's written and sealed," Shaiman says. "So write your own script instead of letting other people write it after you're gone. In fact, don't just *write* it, *live* it while you're alive!"

Curate the Heirlooms That Will Revive Family Memories

Tears sprang to Denise Levenick's eyes as she told the story of one of her favorite family heirlooms: a brooch that frames a tiny picture of her aunt, who was born in 1909, which was taken when she was 4.[16]

Her grandmother lost the little girl in a vicious custody battle and didn't get to raise her. Much later, the aunt became an important advocate for Levenick, supporting her wishes to attend college at a time when her father "thought girls shouldn't go." Even a small trinket like this has the power to tell many stories about multiple generations of a family.

An author and the proprietor of the familycurator.com, Levenick has a mission to help others maintain and pass along the heirlooms and mementos of their family's legacy.

Though scrapbooks, quilts, photographs, hope chests, and other treasures can long outlive their mortal owners, poor storage or handling may destroy them. The memories attached to them can also vanish, erasing their meaning and turning them into objects with no special relevance.

Here's how to help ensure that your personal and family treasures retain their sentimental value.

Document why they're important. Just like you're passing along your personal stories to your descendants, do the same for your mementos' stories,

Levenick says. Write a detailed description of each keepsake, including information such as:

- Where you bought it or who gave it to you
- The name of the company that made it
- When you acquired it
- Why it is important to you
- If you bought it, how much it cost
- A special story about the item ("This cast-iron skillet still has the original protective coating from when your grandmother seasoned it," or "Dad took me to the toy store that used to be downtown to buy me this baseball glove")

Write these stories in a notebook and attach a photo of the object next to each description, or do this more quickly by cutting and pasting digital photos into a word-processing document on your computer.

Without this information, your family may have no inkling of the importance of these objects after you're gone. Nor may they know whether to protect this stuff, toss it, or put a tag on it for a yard sale. Perhaps more important than losing these items, they'd also lose family memories they might have treasured later.

Start rescuing fragile heirlooms now. If some of your family memories are captured on VHS videotapes from the 1980s and '90s, be aware that the clock is ticking on their survival, Levenick warns. Transfer them to a more durable type of storage like a DVD sooner rather than later. (You can find many companies online that provide this service.)

Similarly, some kinds of photo albums can damage the pictures they contain, she says. If you have photos that are valuable enough to pass along, put them in archival-quality albums to protect them.

While you're at it, check whether you have important keepsakes baking in your attic, freezing in your shed, or moldering in your basement. If you do, move them to a place that's safe from the elements, mice, insects, and mildew.

Document your photos, too. Speaking of photographs, "loose pictures are the *worst*," Levenick laughs. If you want your kids or grandkids to appreciate your family's visual history, don't leave them a storage container stuffed with hundreds of unlabeled pictures.

Sort your photos into albums or scrapbooks, and leave plenty of space next to each photo so you can write the names of the people, where they were, what year it was, and a brief story about what was happening, she suggests.

Bring in other family experts. If you're keeping a trove of family heirlooms in storage, it's a good idea to let other family members look at it.

Levenick inherited a trunk of items from her grandmother, a well-traveled and colorful sort who was born in 1890 and was married five times to four husbands. Levenick knew about its existence for decades before she could get her hands on it. But by that time, many of the people who could have told her about the significance of the treasures in the chest were gone. Thus, so were the stories of these objects.

Take a look at memorabilia you've inherited to see if you need to collect their stories from any elders who are still surviving. Let your extended family look at this stuff, too. Your home museum may be holding heirlooms that would be meaningful to the life story of an aunt, uncle, cousin, or other relative.

If you're going to inherit family heirlooms from parents or grandparents in the future, it's also wise to ask them to record the important details about these objects. Or visit them in person and share a storytelling session about these mementos.

Heirlooms May Be an Important Reminder for You Later

Keeping a record of your prized objects' stories isn't just helpful for your legacy. These notes may benefit *you* someday, Denise Levenick, proprietor of The Family Curator Web site, says.

If you ever lose mental clarity due to a stroke, dementia, or old age, these heirlooms can provide important cues to help you recall past events. If your loved ones know the significance of certain items, they may be more likely to show them to you.

LIVE WELL, DIE HAPPY EXERCISES
Chapter 8

1. Walk around your house with a notebook and find five items that remind you of important stories from your past that would be relevant and entertaining for your loved ones. Jot down the significance of these objects, and tell a few of the stories the next time you see a family member who should hear them.

2. What kind of future would you desire for your spouse or partner, kids, and other important people in your life after you're gone? Start collecting these thoughts on paper, which will help you complete your ethical will when you're ready.

3. Think about a skill you could teach someone, or a personal strength you could show someone how to develop. If you keep it to yourself, it will die with you. But if you share it with others, it will become a part of you that lives on. Make a specific plan—with a deadline—to teach it to someone else, and let your loved ones know how you're sharing this part of your legacy.

Part 4

NOW, ON TO THAT "DYING HAPPY" PART

The subject that concludes this book can be avoided no longer. The rest of it is about dying. Us dying, other people dying, sudden deaths, and gradual deaths.

Are you ready?

Have the experts' advice and everyday people's experiences prepared you to approach a discussion about death with openness and curiosity?

In our own lives, we can't avoid the death that comes at the end, either. But we can change how we think about it. When we deny it, refuse to look at it, or pull our loved ones into a heavy silence about it, we allow death to control some of the most precious time of our life.

But we can instead explore death. We can share conversations about it. We can prepare for it so that when we approach it, we do so more on our own terms. We can face it alongside our loved ones, friends, doctors, and the rest of our supporters working as a team.

So, maybe this last section isn't just about dying, after all. Perhaps it's all about discovering new elements of living well . . . for a very important reason.

CHAPTER 9

Coping with Death When It Arrives for Others

For 2 weeks after September 11, 2001, grief counselor Patti Anewalt, PhD, and her colleagues worked to comfort families facing the aftermath of the crash of Flight 93 in Shanksville, Pennsylvania.[1]

Some of the 40 passengers and crew on board had confronted the hijackers who had taken over the jet and flown it off course.[2] Unlike the three other hijacked flights that crashed into densely populated cities that morning, this jet plunged at 563 miles per hour into an empty field near the town.

The heroism of those aboard quickly became an important detail in the nation's retelling of the 9-11 story, and the field now contains a national memorial.

Shortly after that dark day, grieving family members and friends "came to the crash site, and we gave them vials of soil from where their loved ones went down. They were so proud that their loved ones kept the plane from going where it was heading. That was so meaningful and important to them," says Dr. Anewalt, director of the Pathways Center for Grief and Loss in Mount Joy,

Pennsylvania, and a board member of the Association for Death Education and Counseling.

Throughout this book, you've read about the value of *meaning,* such as using it to support your purpose on Earth or direct how you'll spend your time. Experts are becoming increasingly aware that finding meaning in your loss can also help you process your grief after someone close to you dies.

One summer afternoon, I spoke with a leading proponent of meaning in grief, Robert Neimeyer, PhD, a psychology professor at the University of Memphis, while he enjoyed a sandwich and a stroll around his neighborhood.

I found him quite cheery, though his university's magazine once said he "has every reason to be the saddest man . . . on campus." As he told the reporter, his life's work—and I suspect his personal mission statement—is "to help people put their lives back together after a tragedy."[3]

Before we meet our own death, virtually all of us will lose someone we care about. You may already know such grief if you've lost a child, spouse, parent, or close friend. If you haven't yet experienced such a loss (I haven't at this point in my life), now is a good time to learn a little about grief.

You may be carrying some misconceptions about how it works, how it feels, and what we might hope to accomplish from it. Also, you may not realize that people can discover new strengths while grieving, or that their outlook can change in a positive way over the course of a very bleak time.

We'll rejoin Dr. Neimeyer momentarily. But first, a primer on grief.

Grief 101

For starters, let's review a few definitions. Bereavement, grief, and mourning are often used interchangeably when we talk about death. But these words describe different issues.

Some experts define *bereavement* as "the objective situation of having lost someone significant through death." This is the unwanted event at the beginning: Someone you care about has died.[4] *Grief* is your personal reaction to this death, with all of the internal feelings and emotions it brings. *Mourning,* by one common meaning, is your public display of grief (think memorial services, wearing black, and showing culturally expected behaviors).

Though you can grieve other kinds of losses, for the rest of this chapter, let's use the word *grief* to mean your response to the death of a loved one.

Grief is an individual process. You may be under the impression that we all travel in an orderly procession through the five stages of grief that society tells us to expect: denial and isolation, anger, bargaining, depression, and acceptance. You enter the first stage feeling terrible and emerge from the end okay again, right?

Elisabeth Kübler-Ross, MD, discussed these stages as part of people's response to their own impending death in her landmark 1969 book *On Death and Dying*. From there, the public came to apply these stages to grieving for other people.

"I think most people do still think of Dr. Kübler-Ross and those five stages. Quite frankly, I think there are a lot of professional counselors who are still under that impression," says Elizabeth Doughty Horn, PhD, associate professor of counseling at Idaho State University in Meridian. "But honestly, that's very far away from where we are now."[5]

These days, experts regard grief as an individualized experience, she says. Everyone takes their own path through it. One method of viewing the different ways that people grieve is the "adaptive grieving styles" concept described by researchers Kenneth Doka and Terry Martin.

Picture a sliding scale. On one end are so-called *intuitive grievers*. They feel intense emotions related to their loss and tend to show them publicly. Someone with this grieving style may feel that "I need to cry a lot; I need to talk with lots of people about that loss, say a grief support group; and I need to have an emotional outward expression," Dr. Horn says. If you associate particular responses with different areas of your body, intuitive grieving may feel centered around your heart. Also, this is stereotypically considered a more female type of grieving, she says.

On the other end of the scale are *instrumental grievers*. This type of grief occurs more in the head than the heart. These individuals may try to think their way through their grief, approaching it as a problem to be solved. This emotionally cool, logical approach is more stereotypically associated with men.

Intuitive grieving style   **Instrumental grieving style**

Most of us fall somewhere between the two, and women and men can display grief at either end, Dr. Horn says. But characteristics of either grieving style may look "wrong" to friends, coworkers, or even family members. They may think that someone who's grieving too openly, intensely, or for too long needs to "move on," or that someone else who's too detached, reserved, and calm is in denial.

"That's a big part of what grief counseling is these days: allowing people to have that natural experience and expression. We also educate them that their loved one who's not doing it the way they want can still be having a healthy response, even if it looks very different from their own," Dr. Horn says.

Grief isn't about "moving on" or forgetting. The grieving process doesn't have to let you leave your loss in the past. Instead, it can help you develop a new type of relationship with the missing person. Grief expert Thomas Attig, PhD, has written that grieving is, "in part, our making the transition from loving persons who are present to loving them in their absence."[6]

A word for this shift is "adaptation," Dr. Horn says. "In the past we saw that with grief, you were trying to do all these things to find closure, to find an end to grief. That thinking has shifted more to, 'I'm adapting to my life without this person.' That adaptation will continue for the rest of your life in some regards, certainly in lesser degrees later on, and it looks very different for each individual," she says.

"You're trying to create a new connection to this person who is no longer physically in your world. That connection is a more personal and meaningful one. I'm not talking about obsessively keeping shrines or trying to maintain the same type of relationship, but you might talk to them, feel their presence at times, and feel connected and close in some way," she says.

Grieving is a form of "remembering well," says Dan Moseley, DMin, Indianapolis author and former pastor and seminary professor. "A lot of people say that to grieve well, you have to forget the past and move on. I say you have to remember it until it becomes human." Some people idealize their lost loved one, some dwell on their shortcomings, and some remember them as a complex, *real* person, he says.

"We do not forget the past. It exists within us. The question becomes how we integrate it into the world we live in. If we do not give the past a voice, it'll scream out at some point in our lives and demand attention," he says.

Many variables can affect your grief. The depth and length of the grief you feel can vary based on several factors, including:[7]

- Your age
- The amount of emotional support surrounding you
- The type of relationship you had with the deceased, such as parent, child, or spouse
- The emotional closeness or distance of the relationship
- Whether the death was expected or a surprise
- Whether the death was due to a natural cause or some other event, such as murder, suicide, or an accident

Grief comes in several forms. You can have *anticipatory* grief when a loved one is approaching death. It doesn't necessarily help you expel your sad feelings ahead of time, as if you have a battery charged with a preset amount of grief. But it may help motivate you to take care of any unfinished business before death arrives, like reconnecting with an estranged loved one, or asking for forgiveness or offering it.[8]

Typically, after the death, the grief begins in an *acute* form, according to Katherine Shear, MD, a grief expert and professor of psychiatry at Columbia University in New York City. Your emotions, which run the gamut from anger to anxiety to depression, can feel overwhelming. You're likely to feel a deep yearning for the departed loved one, withdraw from your usual activities, and have trouble believing this person is gone. Your blood pressure and stress hormones may rise. You may have a sort of hallucination in which you see or hear the departed. Your risk of heart attack goes up, as does your risk of another potentially serious condition called broken heart syndrome, which has similar symptoms.[9,10]

But during this time, you can also have good thoughts and feelings about your missing loved one. You may feel happy about the good times and silly moments you shared.

After a period of time—often by 6 months—people typically start transitioning into *integrated grief,* which lasts the rest of their lives. The sense of sadness and of missing the loved one lessens. The grief no longer disrupts daily activities so severely. People can again feel happiness, and they can turn their thoughts back to the business of living. However, intense episodes of sadness and yearning for the departed loved one often continue to flare up around special occasions, like holidays and particularly happy or sad events.

But sometimes, people don't make the transition to integrated grief. They may feel "stuck" in the depths of acute grief. In some cases, this is called *complicated grief.* According to Dr. Shear, who focuses on complicated grief, research has shown that it affects nearly 7 percent of bereaved people. The main symptoms are similar to those of acute grief: a deep longing for the missing person; trouble accepting the death; feelings of guilt or anger; numbness; and isolation from others (in part because friends and family may drift away).

Complicated grief is particularly common in parents after the death of a child and in individuals after the death of a romantic partner. Research has found that older women are particularly prone to experiencing it.

Other factors that may make you more likely to suffer from complicated grief or its symptoms after the death of a loved one include:

- Challenging interactions with medical providers around the time of the individual's death

- Trouble accepting the loved one's illness before the death

- Conflict at the end of life within a family that's usually more agreeable

We'll talk about navigating around these end-of-life threats in coming chapters, and also how to make the best use of hospice care, which may lower survivors' risk of complicated grief.

Telling Stories and Finding Meaning May Help You Process Your Grief

In an academic paper published in 2014, Dr. Neimeyer shared the story of a soon-to-be retired grandfather whose hopes and plans were overturned when he learned that his son and grandson were missing after a boating accident. Their bodies were not found until months later.[11]

Though religious, the man "contended with the image of a universe and a God made suddenly more random or cruel than he had imagined, precipitating a spiritual struggle that distanced him from his once-important church community. And practically he was forced to rewrite the hoped-for script of his life in a changed family and a changed landscape," Dr. Neimeyer wrote. This process required refashioning his connection to his two lost loved ones.

The man began discussing boating safety in schools and media appearances. He also persuaded the park service to erect kiosks that offered free life jackets on loan next to a picture of his son and grandson. In short, he shared their stories and discovered new meaning, both to give his own life structure and to provide an explanation for his loved ones' deaths.

You can find plenty of examples of grieving survivors taking a similar approach.

After his son, Adam, was kidnapped and murdered in 1981, hotel developer John Walsh cofounded the National Center for Missing and Exploited Children. He later focused a national spotlight on fugitives as host of the long-running *America's Most Wanted* television program.[12]

In addition, dozens of laws and acts across the country are named after children who died, in the hopes of protecting other kids and their families from tragedy.[13] Every time the broadcast media deliver an AMBER Alert for a missing child, they're also commemorating an abducted 9-year-old Texas girl named Amber. Mothers Against Drunk Driving began in the bedroom of a

13-year-old girl, shortly after she was struck and killed by a hit-and-run driver.[14]

Dr. Neimeyer told me that he sees grieving "as a process of reaffirming or rebuilding a world of meaning that has been challenged by loss." Our stories—the same tools that help us *explain* how we fit into our families, *pass along* wisdom, and *anticipate* what happens to us after we die—can also help us in these moments.

"We're storytelling beings. Unsurprisingly, when we're confronted by great adversity, we attempt to make a story out of it, a narrative that makes sense of the experience. I think that narrative effort really has two points of focus," Dr. Neimeyer says. "One is on attempting to process the story of our loved one's death to grapple with the issues of what happened: 'What kind of cosmos could allow my child to die at the age of 2 of mysterious causes?' or 'What would lead my partner to take his life by suicide?'

"But we also are looking for the meaning of that death for our *own* lives: 'Who am I now that I'm no longer a mother to a living child?'" he says. "What is my life about now that I'm no longer married to this person who's been my partner all of those years?"

The bereaved survivor may need to learn how to tell the loved one's story so the death doesn't overshadow the life, and how to preserve memories that "can serve as a source of inspiration and maybe companionship," he says. "We're looking for a way to maintain their relevance to our life rather than eliminate it."

But sometimes, people may need to walk away from their memories and *not* carry forward the missing person's voice, such as in the case of an abusive or hypercritical parent or spouse who's died, Dr. Neimeyer says.

Reaching Out to Others Can Be Helpful—But Not Everyone Needs It

The modern awareness that everyone grieves differently has brought more acceptance that for some people, this period just isn't so, well, grief-stricken.

People tend to follow different trajectories in their grief, according to George Bonanno, PhD, professor of clinical psychology at Columbia

Take Care When Putting Messages in Time Capsules

The public radio program *This American Life* told a fascinating true story about how messages from beyond the grave might help grieving loved ones, but they can also have unintended consequences.

As she was dying of breast cancer, Elizabeth Gee wrote a series of letters to her then 16-year-old daughter, Rebekah. The plan was for Rebekah to unseal a new letter on her birthday for the next 12 years. She'd have another to open on her wedding day. Sometimes, the letters offered a sense of connection and guidance. "When I decided I didn't have the confidence to go to medical school and I wasn't going to do it, the letter that year basically said, 'You need to find ethical expression in your work,'" Rebekah told the radio program. "For most of college, I think I had this enormous sense of purpose that I had a responsibility to do something meaningful, both to me and to other people." Eventually, she became the head of Louisiana's Department of Health.

On the other hand, the arrival of new letters (her father was responsible for sending them) could dredge up sadness for her loss and at times, guilt. Her mother urged her to commit to the Mormon church and marry a fellow believer. But Rebekah was already drifting away.

The final letter for her wedding day, which occurred in an Episcopal church, vanished in the mail. Just 18 months later, her husband was killed in a traffic accident. If she'd received ongoing messages from him, they might have interfered with her ability to adapt to her new life, she said.

Today, e-mail services make it easy for you to store messages that go out after you die. If you do this, keep in mind that your audience will be in a new stage of life, and they may be heading in directions you can't predict now.

Your messages might inspire your loved ones, or they may awaken their grief. They might sound comforting—or pushy. And you won't be there to help the readers sort through any unintended fallout your messages cause. So if you want to keep talking after you depart, choose your words with care.

University in New York City. One of these is a trajectory marked by *resilience.* Following the death, such people may have a moderate spike in distress and depression that quickly subsides over the next few months. This is in contrast to having higher initial levels of depression and grief that diminish over time (usually a year or two) or that remain chronically high.[15] Not everyone needs some sort of grief therapy after losing a loved one, it seems.

However, working through your grief with someone else—such as a mental health professional or a support group of fellow bereaved individuals—may be advisable in some cases. If you're more of an intuitive griever (the heartfelt emotional style), grief counseling that gives you space to talk and cry might be particularly helpful, Dr. Horn says.

You may be able to find a support group in your area that's specific to your type of loss, Dr. Anewalt says. For example, her organization offers groups for people who've lost a child, a spouse, or a parent, or any loved one to suicide. One common benefit from participating in a support group is that over time, as the bereaved listen to other members' experiences, they often realize the progress they're making on their own grief journey, she says.

Working one-on-one with a therapist may also help you find meaning in your loss. This approach may be particularly useful for people with the more thinking-oriented instrumental grieving style, Dr. Horn says. According to Dr. Neimeyer, therapists can use a number of techniques to help bereaved people seek meaning through storytelling, such as journaling and other writing exercises.

If your loved one received care from a hospice before dying, the hospice organization may offer bereavement education and counseling. Medicare provides for hospice-based bereavement services to families before their loved one's death and for up to a year afterward.[16, 17]

A mental health professional may also be helpful in treating complicated grief. In a 2016 study published in *JAMA Psychiatry,* Dr. Shear and colleagues divided 395 bereaved adults into four groups. Some went through a 16-session therapy program designed for complicated grief and also took either the antidepressant citalopram or a placebo. The two other groups took only the antidepressant or the placebo, with no therapy.[18]

Those who went through only the therapy were more likely to have a good response compared to those who used only the placebo. That suggests the therapy alone was helpful. But among the people who went through therapy, those who also took the antidepressant had a significantly greater improvement in their symptoms of depression.

Major Depression, PTSD May Strike Alongside Grief

Grief is not the same as major depression. However, grief *is* a common trigger for episodes of major depression in people of all ages.[19]

Mental health professionals can't always tell when a grieving person also has depression that needs to be treated. Symptoms that grief and major depression can share include sadness and a desire to withdraw socially.

However, other factors can help a professional distinguish between the two. During grief, your low mood tends to become less intense over time, with occasional "pangs" when you think about the person who died. But in major depression, the low mood tends to persist. Also, you're likely to have feelings of worthlessness during major depression, but not grief.

"The question is not so much whether a recently bereaved individual is depressed *or* grieving; but rather whether or not the person is grieving *and* also has a major depressive episode triggered by their loss, which accompanies and exacerbates the grief," a group of experts wrote in a 2014 issue of *Current Psychiatry Reports.*

Your risk of post-traumatic stress disorder (PTSD) may also be higher after the death of a loved one, especially if the death was due to suicide, an accident, or an act of violence, or if you have complicated grief. (On the other hand, if you already had PTSD before the death, you may be more likely to develop complicated grief.)

The Mayo Clinic recommends contacting your doctor if you're depressed. Do the same if possible PTSD symptoms may be affecting your life, such as distressing memories, hopelessness, severe guilt, and trouble concentrating. If you're having suicidal thoughts, call 911, a suicide hotline (such as 800-273-TALK), your doctor, or a mental health professional.[20, 21]

Always remember that everything is temporary. The clothing fashions and TV shows you enjoy, your job, your appearance, and your health will all change. Even the beach you visited or the mountain you summited on vacation will, given enough time, vanish.

So, too, will the people you love.

When they do, you'll grieve on your own timeline and in the way that is right for you, Dr. Horn says. It's no one else's place to tell you that you're doing it right or wrong. Over time, you will likely be able to integrate your loss into your daily life. Odds are good that you'll come up with a meaning for why the death happened and a meaning for the new life you're writing for yourself. But if you need help with the grieving process—or related depression or anxiety—it's out there.

"There's a deep wisdom in why this process only unfolds a little bit at a time. I realized a long time ago that if we grieved in 3 or 4 days, we'd burn out biochemically," long-time Colorado grief educator Kim Mooney told me.

"You tell your story to someone, and every time you tell it, it's like everything shifts a little bit. That's how it settles into place within us. Some people *don't* talk about it, but as they move along, their story shifts, and at some point down the road, they have a new life that grows around the story. At some point we integrate this brokenheartedness. It's still there, but we grow bigger muscles around it," she says.

LIVE WELL, DIE HAPPY EXERCISES
Chapter 9

1. List three difficult losses you've had to face. These could be the death of someone close to you or the loss of something else important, like a job or a marriage. What resources helped you get through these hardships? How did your outlook about the losses change over time, and what are your thoughts on them now? _____

_____

_____

_____

_____

_____

_____

2. Do you know where you could find support for bereavement grief, such as a counselor, therapist, or support group, in your community? Go online to see what sorts of resources are available in your area. (If you've started volunteering at a local hospice, you could also ask around there.)

3. Have you ever observed someone grieving a death? Was their style more intuitive or instrumental? Did they find some sort of meaning to explain the death or its place in their changed world? How long did the acute phase of their grief seem to last? How do they seem now, compared to how they were before the death? _____

_____

_____

_____

_____

_____

_____

CHAPTER 10

Live as if Death Might Surprise You (Because It Might)

A great deal of effort goes into tracking how we die.

In government agencies, universities, and other organizations, fatality reports continually roll in, and the statisticians and actuaries carefully compile and analyze the data. Tucked away in all those columns of numbers is a fact that will launch this chapter: Men are much more likely to die in traffic accidents than women. Apparently we drive more miles, which simply exposes us to more risk. But we also speed more frequently and click our seat belts into place less often.[1]

Each year, more than twice as many men as women die on the road. The numbers are even more dramatic in bicycle-versus-auto accidents. In 2014, 637 male cyclists were killed, compared to just 81 females.

Let us now turn our attention to two men—Jose Hernando and Chad Moor—whose deaths are now tallied in these statistics. While motor vehicles caused their lives to end, their legacies endure today in unexpected but meaningful ways, with the help of the loved ones they left behind.

At 44, Hernando still maintained a fitness level that a younger man could envy, his body honed and streamlined from participating on an amateur cycling team in Seattle. With a job as a computer engineer, a preteen daughter, and a son about to start kindergarten, he was fully engaged in a busy phase of his life. Money had been tight at times since they moved into their new home, but he and his wife, Chanel Reynolds, were getting by.[2]

On a training ride in June 2009, he collided with a van. The paramedics who arrived at the scene didn't anticipate that he'd make it to the hospital alive, given the severity of the injuries to his spine and brain.

In 2000, Chad Moor and his wife, Carolyn, were a 36-year-old couple running a successful Florida interior design firm with 50 employees. Valentine's Day found them in a romantic mood, as it did every year.[3]

They hired a babysitter for their two young daughters and—after a stop in the bedroom—headed out for dinner and a stroll around the lake in a wooded park in downtown Orlando. Carolyn snapped a selfie of them together to preserve the moment.

They didn't return home together at the end of the evening. A hit-and-run driver slammed into their car, ejecting Chad from the vehicle. Carolyn was uninjured, but Chad remained unconscious for 2 days before he died. Like *that,* she says, their life together was over.

Most of us—men or women—aren't going to die suddenly like Jose and Chad. Instead, you can probably expect to see your death coming well before it arrives. A doctor may treat the problem that eventually kills you, or at least contributes to your death, for months or years. Before death comes, you'll probably have time to put your affairs in order and have important conversations with your loved ones.

Of the most common causes of death, accidents, heart attacks, strokes, and suicides are the only entries that generally come as a jolt for you and your loved ones.[4] Altogether, these account for only about 16 percent of deaths. Even when you include dying from homicide, drug overdose, dissected aorta, and surgical treatment that goes bad, the fact remains: Death is more likely to slowly walk up to you in full view than to surprise you from behind.

But still, our connection to life could end at any time. Like *that.*

So live as if death isn't going to pay you the courtesy of advance notice. Live as if it'll surprise you from behind.

If you don't, the days after you depart may be much harder for your loved ones to navigate. The tasks they have to manage may drain already-scarce resources. Or the legacy that you created may forever bear a blemish because of one missed conversation. An unresolved hurt within someone you care about could grow into a lingering sore spot.

All because you were going to take care of these needs on some future day, and it never came.

Get It Together While the Getting's Good

When she reached the emergency room after Jose's accident, Chanel Reynolds immediately realized that her life, as she knew it, was over.

"It was clear that no matter what happened next, if he lived or died, we'd basically be totally screwed," she says.

She paused a moment to acknowledge that what she was about to discuss is awkward to put into words, since we're not supposed to talk about how a loved one's death would impact our finances. However, that reluctance is a reason why we *need* to bring it out into the open.

"The injuries to his body were severe, and we weren't certain yet how badly his brain had been injured. My fingers were still crossed that it would be a long physical therapy and years-long recovery for my husband, hoping he'd be able to regain some ability to engage with the world. All of that would cost a lot of money. We had no short-term or long-term disability insurance. We'd stretched to buy a two-income family home."

If that happened, she thought, she'd have to sell the house. Her son would have to change schools. She realized that Jose's health insurance would eventually run out, and "then we'd slowly go bankrupt, and it would be incredibly hard on everyone," she says.

"But the ER doctor kept saying he could die any second. The last thing I wanted was to lose my husband. Then I'd be living as a single mom of a young child and stepdaughter trying to make ends meet by myself in a life I couldn't afford."

Circumstances decided that Reynolds would be going down the second route. The young widow found that some of the advance planning the couple had done made her first steps as a single mom a little easier, like the "small but helpful life insurance policy" they had bought when their son was born.

But the planning they *didn't* complete led to a stampede of frustrations that made Chanel's transition much, much harder.

"When I was at the hospital, they handed me my husband's phone, but I didn't have the four-number password to get into it and call his family. I spent *hours* trying to guess the password. That was a lot of additional noise and stress I couldn't handle at that moment. Also, our wills and living wills were drafted and had been sitting in my e-mail inbox for 6 months. They were not signed or notarized, which made them not worth the paper they *would* have been printed on if I'd printed them!" she says.

The would-have-been-preventable hassles continued in the following months. Merely accessing their accounts with banks, insurance companies, utilities, and other services required her to spend "hundreds of hours on the phone with various 'I'm sorry for your loss' departments trying to track stuff down," she says.

Eventually, Reynolds poured the knowledge she learned from the couple's experience into a Web site called Get Your Shit Together, which has since become GYST.com. Its mission is to educate people on the basic financial and legal planning they should do just in case death suddenly interrupts their lives. (In retrospect, she admits, the full name tends to present difficulties when she holds programs for worship congregations.)

Some of her recommendations will require 5 minutes. Others will take longer. Nonetheless, start doing them now—which is a moment you know you have—rather than waiting until later, which is less certain.

Share your passwords. A growing number of your daily tasks may flow through the Internet now. Odds are good that you pay your mortgage online, track bills through your smartphone, and maintain your social connections with Facebook.

Accessing all these accounts would be difficult, at best, for loved ones who don't have your user name and password. Bills could fall between the cracks, or your family could miss time-sensitive deadlines that cost money.

So create a central place to put your user names and passwords, either in an online password manager or on a sheet of paper, if you're concerned about privacy. Keep the list secure, but be sure your spouse, partner, or anyone else who might need this information knows where to find it.

Every time you choose a user name and password in your day-to-day life, take a moment to jot them down on this new record. Don't forget to also write down any login information that you've asked your computer to automatically fill in for particular Web sites, as well as your access information for your phone, streaming TV services, and other devices.

Get enough insurance to build a bridge. Buying life insurance can be a particularly unnerving task, which I think is due in part to the warnings you may find online that urge you to purchase a small fortune's worth of protection. "If I insured myself for as much as I really wanted, it would be about $1,000 a month. Almost no one can afford that, so I carry enough to cover the kids if anything happens to me," Reynolds says.

Her advice is to get at least enough to provide your spouse or partner with "a bridge between the old life and the new one." Your partner may need to take time away from work to deal with grief, sort out household business, and get moving again. So "buy them enough time that they don't have to make stress-induced decisions. Those never go well," she says.

Sit down with your household budget and figure out:

- Your monthly expenses
- How much of those expenses your income covers
- How many expenses would go away if you died (perhaps your car, and its payment, and part of the grocery bill)
- How many new expenses your death would create (like your funeral)

Then plan how many months'—or years'—worth of cushion you want your partner to have, and purchase life insurance accordingly. If you can afford enough for your partner to retire and your kids to go to college debt-free, then by all means buy more insurance. But at least cover this minimum.

While you're at it, buy disability insurance if you don't already have it and your family depends on your income. If an illness or injury were to leave you out of work for a few months before you die, your family would have an added layer of protection.

Create a savings fund. Reynolds agrees with the wisdom of setting aside enough savings to cover 6 months' worth of your household bills. A survey released in 2016 by Bankrate.com found that 28 percent of Americans don't have *any* emergency savings, and another 18 percent don't have enough to cover 3 months' worth of expenses.[5]

Building this reserve may take some time, but you might find that the expenses you cut from your budget don't make a detectable difference in your life.

An approach that works well in my household is to ask before each purchase, "Am I going to be using this in 30 days, or at least have happy memories of it?" If an impulse buy is just going to disappear into the clutter of your home or you're not going to notice the difference if you buy only three $5 pints of ice cream instead of four, then why buy it?

Also, think about whether spending your money on an endless flow of momentary impulses truly supports the long-term plans you've been creating.

Prepare your important paperwork. If you were to succumb to a rapid illness or sudden injury tomorrow, three documents could help determine your quality of life in your final moments—and your loved ones' quality of life once you're gone, Reynolds says.

A WILL. Your will lets you decide who gets your money and property and who will raise your kids to adulthood. No one else can make these decisions as well as you can, but without your wishes in a legal document, court authorities who don't know you may have to try.

A trust is another method of distributing your assets that you may want to use instead of a will or in addition to it. Whichever you choose, you'll need to select a trustworthy, responsible adult to act as the executor of the will or as the trustee of the trust. This is the person who makes sure your wishes are carried out per your directions—even if some of your family members aren't happy with your decisions. Choose with care.

A LIVING WILL. Also called an advance directive, this is different from the kind of will that specifies who should get your dining room furniture. Your advance directive stipulates the type of life-sustaining interventions you would want a doctor to provide if you were unconscious in a life-threatening situation.

At the end, Reynolds asked for her husband to be taken off life support, since it was only prolonging his death. Because the heads of the hospital's neurology and palliative care departments had told her that Jose had no chance of recovering, she felt that this was the right call. Still, it was the hardest decision she'd ever made.

"If in that week, he'd woken up for half a second, or fluttered his eyelid or done anything to give me any hope, even though I knew he would never want to live like this, I don't know how I could have done it," she says.

"The temptation is to think about what *you* want and how desperate *you* are to have that person get better." In these circumstances, your advance directive can serve as a guiding star for your loved ones that says, "Here is the gift I can give to you with clarity so you don't have to worry or wonder. You just have to do for me what I can't do for myself," she says.

You'll find a detailed guide in Chapter 11 on how to create your advance directive and then talk to your loved ones about it. Just remember that this document isn't only potentially useful in the distant future. You and your loved ones might need it sooner than any of you would like.

DURABLE POWER OF ATTORNEY. This legal tool gives your approval to someone else to make important decisions on your behalf if you are not capable of doing so. Despite the name, this representative doesn't need to be an attorney—but they need to be someone you trust.

You'll also read more about this document in the next chapter. Create it without delay.

If It's Worth Saying or Doing, Then Say It or Do It Today

Carolyn Moor was able to sidestep some of the early difficulties that Reynolds faced, due in part to some well-timed planning.

The untimely death of 42-year-old golfer Payne Stewart—who lived in their city—made Moor and her husband, Chad, realize that even in their midthirties, they needed to do some advance planning. (Authorities believe the jet crash that took Stewart's life was due to a loss of cabin pressure that caused the pilots to lose consciousness.)[6]

"We were on clients' private jets all the time. I refused to fly on a plane with my husband until we had a will. We had two small children at home and the design firm, and I told him, 'If both of us go down, it'll be catastrophic for a lot of people.' I didn't know that 4 months later he was going to die."

Before their Valentine's Day car accident, they had also gone through their bills, their household paperwork, and "the infrastructure of our relationship" together, so Moor had a handle on their personal and business finances, she says.

She continued working in interior design for another 15 years, but now her mission is Modern Widows Club, a national advocacy and education organization that she founded in 2011. She spoke with me about another kind of investment that you can provide for your loved ones to draw upon later: the gift of connectedness.

The Moors' usual tradition on Valentine's Day was "to replay the past, to really soak in all the joy of what it felt like when we met, and to replay the story of 'when you asked me to marry you,' then the wedding, and the rest of the timeline of our life together."

So, when she thinks of their last evening together—but many of the evenings before, as well—she has plenty of fond memories to replay.

The time to create your memories is *now*. Supply your loved ones with a steady flow of stories, conversations, in-jokes, traditions, and daily reminders of the feelings you have for them.

In short, while you're alive, *be* alive! If you were to die next week, these are the ways your loved ones could be remembering you next month.

History may someday tell our descendants that we lost more good years of life in the early 2000s to handheld electronic devices than to any disease. It's hard to be mindful of the present moment when the tiny screen continually beckons you to log in and disappear.

So whenever you have an opportunity to focus your full attention on your spouse, your kids, or your other loved ones, put away your electronic distractions. Set your tablet in a drawer and lock it. Stack your phones on the table, and the first person to pick one up has to do the least-favorite household chore. Then just *listen* with your full attention. (This may take some practice at first.)

"Find a way to truly be present when you're with someone. I mean, that's *it*. I've heard so many people talk about how they wish they'd 'paid attention' or 'had that conversation.' It really becomes very simple: All of those little moments become your legacy," Moor says.

Well-Planned Paperwork Made Grieving Daughter's Job Easier

The first time Amy Oravec's father introduced her to The Binder, she wanted nothing to do with it. But much later, it turned out to be quite the helpful and well-informed friend.

"It was a huge green notebook that contained everything from his and my mom's will to the selling price of the house—including which Realtor to call—to his life insurance and the lawyer I should contact," says Oravec, a medical editor in Philadelphia. Her father had even outfitted The Binder with color-coded tabs and an index. In a side pocket, she found a note that said, "If you are reading this now, I have croaked."

She says that "every time he took it out to show me, I waved him away. I didn't want to talk about it, since he was never going to die." Given her father's durability in the face of multiple maladies, that wasn't an unreasonable expectation.

Malcolm Orloff, PhD, was a chemist turned business executive. After he had an open-heart procedure to replace a valve at age 57, his doctors recommended another major surgery to repair an aneurysm in his aorta, the large artery exiting the heart.

Dr. Orloff declined, preferring to watch and wait. He later

Reynolds shares a similar sentiment. Don't just seize the day—seize the moment.

"Get your shit together in your life! Finish the unfinished. Clean up your business. Return your neighbor's rake. Talk to your dad. Just do the things that we're afraid to do," she says.

"I miss my husband dearly. I was and still am in some ways devastated from his loss. But he and I were *clean.* I can live each day knowing that there wasn't anything left unsaid. We had a successful—not perfect, but *successful*—marriage. I don't have to carry around guilt or shame with me."

developed prostate cancer, which didn't initially seem aggressive. Plus, his doctor suspected that his aneurysm would kill him first. So he didn't get treatment for the cancer, either.

"His bankers told me that each time he came in to see them, he said, 'This could be the last time you see me.' This went on for 10 years." But eventually Dr. Orloff succumbed to the cancer at age 75. In her bereavement, Oravec turned to The Binder.

"In my panic over his death, I am sure I wouldn't have even been able to think clearly. It was so much work for me as the executrix of the estate, and getting everything finished took a year and a half, which is really not that bad. For that I thank The Binder," she says.

"I do wish we'd talked about my dad's illness/finances/inheritance/ funeral seriously, and I now realize it would have given him peace of mind," she says. But he never mentioned that he was actually, truly dying, and they hadn't had a history of many serious talks.

"If I could advise anyone on this matter, I would say if your parents— or anyone—want to talk to you about finances or death, please sit down and listen. You will learn a great deal, and it will make the person feel secure and confident in your abilities. I regret not having had this type of serious talk with my dad because it would have given him reassurance, but in the long run, I did just fine . . . only he didn't know."

Reynolds finished our conversation with a point that you'll see again in the next few pages. Using some of your present moments to square away unfinished business, including your end-of-life wishes, is a remarkable way to embark on many other important discussions.

"After talking to so many people and doing this work for a number of years, it dawned on me that this is not just my story. It's everyone's story. When we do these basic things and share them with the people we need to share them with, it creates a lot of room for having the bigger conversations. In almost every circumstance and with every person I've talked to, it ends up being a happy, joyous, relief-filled conversation and not the hard one we've imagined it to be," she says.

LIVE WELL, DIE HAPPY EXERCISES
Chapter 10

1. Look out for yourself. More than 5 percent of deaths in America are due to injuries from unintentional accidents. These include the bathtub falls, drowsy car crashes, drownings, and firearm mishaps. Very often, such accidents can be prevented. Sometimes heart attacks, strokes, and ruptured aneurysms can, too. So think about ways you might reduce your risk of sudden death. Visit the National Safety Council online (nsc.org) for advice on preventing accidents, and visit your doctor to be screened—and possibly treated—for potential or existing conditions to reduce your risk of medical crises that could strike suddenly.

2. Think about passwords. Did the advice on page 167 about sharing your login information with your spouse make you cringe? *(What if she looked in my phone? What if he had access to that bank account?)* This is a good opportunity to examine your relationship. Would any of your words or actions not stand up to another person's scrutiny? Do you have a lack of trust in your spouse? Perhaps it would be helpful to have a conversation with yourself—and another with your partner—to try to resolve any secrecy or uncertainties in your relationship.

3. Create that ethical will now. Shortly after her husband died, Moor created a lengthy video containing advice and life stories for her daughters, just in case something happened to her, too. You never know when your loved ones might want a heartfelt message from you in your absence. How about creating it now?

Discussing Death with Your Loved Ones

Betty Kramer, PhD, is familiar with the many ways that even a well-meaning family can unravel when a loved one is dying. So when her mother was diagnosed with Stage 4 cancer, she decided to be proactive.

"I knew that a lot of my siblings were very attached to our mother, and her death could destroy them. I said, 'I just want to have a heart-to-heart with you guys. She is going to die, and there's nothing we can do to stop it,'" she told me.[1]

"We have really benefited from her love, and the greatest gift we can give her is to come together and work in harmony to make sure her needs are met. She doesn't want to see us bickering or stressed. So can we think about how to do this in a way so that at the end of the day we can be proud of what we've done? Because this is it. There are no do-overs," she says.

Dr. Kramer, a professor of social work at the University of Wisconsin–Madison, had already experienced a loved one's graceful response to death. Long ago, before leukemia took her 16-year-old brother, he pulled his family in for one-on-one conversations.

"He told me that he knew he was dying, but he was okay with it. He didn't want me to be sad; he said he wanted me to finish college, and he told me what he appreciated about me." (Sound familiar? That's a spoken version of an ethical will.)

Discussing death with your family members isn't necessarily easy. But it is necessary.

Most likely, you're going to need help at the end of your life. You'll probably have a phase, perhaps an extended one, when your physical and mental capabilities are diminished. You may need a caregiver. You may need someone to make very important decisions for you because you can't make them for yourself. That's not an ideal time for your first-ever discussions on life-and-death matters to begin. Nor do you want your family to explode in conflict as you're dying, which is an area of Dr. Kramer's research expertise.

Assuring better outcomes for the end of your life is a task you should begin—you guessed it—*now*.

By starting end-of-life planning today, you may prevent a crisis far in the future. The openness you've encouraged may help you better enjoy your final days on your own terms and may enable your family to navigate this period with greater wellness and peace of mind.

Plus, as you heard at the end of the previous chapter, discussing life and death with your loved ones can make space for a deeper understanding of each other. Honestly, whose relationships couldn't use more of that?

Even if you aren't expecting to die for decades, you should be preparing for it. That's what the rest of this book will help you do. Ideally, this preparation begins with the step described below.

Step 1: Schedule a Conversation

If you want to die well, you must plan for it, says Simon Oczkowski, MD, a critical care physician and end-of-life researcher at McMaster University in Ontario, Canada. This planning requires talking about your eventual death with the people closest to you. What's your version of a "good death"? You need to know the answer to that question, and then they need to know.[2]

"For the patients and their families who come to the intensive care unit (ICU), we can provide high-quality care at the end of life and a dignified, meaningful death," he told me. But a different experience is also available, if you want to consider that option.

"At the other end of the spectrum, some people and their families come in, and it's chaos. They've never thought about death, they've never considered it, and they're grasping at straws until the very end. As a result, they have a very medicalized, undignified death," he says. "I try to steer more toward the former, trying to give people the best death possible when death is inevitable, and avoiding the long, drawn-out, conflict-ridden end-of-life experience that some people have in the ICU."

Opening a discussion with your loved ones about dying can be difficult. It can be awkward. But these conversations will help steer you toward the better outcome that Dr. Oczkowski mentioned, and they "need to take place early and often. We need to normalize having these conversations. It should be considered part of our adult responsibility to have them," says Harriet Warshaw, the executive director of The Conversation Project, which offers guides that can walk you through such discussions.[3]

At their core, these conversations explore the type of medical care you might want during a hypothetical health crisis or at the end of a long illness. They should involve your partner or spouse, and your kids when they're old enough.

"If you're a 45- or 50-year-old, as your kids are approaching young adulthood, start having these conversations before anyone's ill. We want to start early so people have time to become comfortable. It becomes acceptable talk within a family," Warshaw says.

As you get older or your health declines to the point where the idea of dying isn't quite so hypothetical, your end-of-life planning won't be as difficult because you've previously laid the groundwork. (If your fifties are well behind you or you already have an illness that could end your life, making plans now is still a great idea to reduce trouble down the road.)

Think about when a good time to have the initial conversation might arise in the near future, experts at The Conversation Project suggest. At a holiday gathering? The next time you fly out to see an adult child? Or perhaps you'll want to have the talk before an important change, like before your kids move off to college or get married, or while your health is good, if you have a condition that waxes and wanes.[4]

Where's a place that everyone will feel the most relaxed and comfortable? Perhaps it's around the family dinner table, or on a hiking trail, or at the beach, or while everyone's in the minivan on a road trip. (Being in nature or on a long car journey might give you metaphors for your death discussion.)

One way to break the ice is to bring up the illness or death of a celebrity or someone within your family or circle of friends, says Judy Thomas, JD, the CEO of the Coalition for Compassionate Care of California. The organization focuses on improving care during serious illness and at the end of life.[5]

If a death was surprising, you could start the conversation with, "I was just thinking about what if that happened to me." Or if a prominent person used her illness to raise awareness of a disease or to inspire donations to a charitable cause, you could use the news to talk about how you'd like your final days to provide a meaningful and fitting end to your life story.

Late Actor's Eerie Legacy Still Going Strong after 30 Years

Shortly after he died of lung cancer in 1985, actor Yul Brynner reappeared on television seemingly from beyond the grave, fixing the viewer with a piercing gaze while he said, "Now that I'm gone, I tell you, don't smoke." The startling commercial is still circulating online, and it remains one of the most-cited aspects of the actor's legacy.[6]

These conversations won't guarantee that your death will perfectly conform to your every wish, just as avoiding smoking doesn't mean you'll never get lung cancer, or planning a natural childbirth ensures that you'll have one. But talking about your end-of-life wishes is one of the most helpful things you can do to set a course for your desired outcome.

"What we see and hear from people is that when they have had those conversations, it's more likely that their end of life is what they'd hoped for because people were advocating for it, and because someone in the healthcare system knew about it," Warshaw says.

"Even when it's not possible to act on those wishes in totality, if patients and loved ones feel like they've *tried* to act on the wishes, that seems to be just as important. For the people left behind, the feeling that they knew what their loved one wanted and made a good-faith effort helps with the grieving process."

Before you gather your loved ones for The Big Conversation, make sure you know what you're going to tell them. That's the next step.

Step 2: Put Your Important Values in Writing

In his excellent book *Being Mortal,* surgeon and author Atul Gawande, MD, told the story of a professor with a growth in his spinal cord who was weighing whether or not to have major surgery. He could crunch a lot of numbers for his decision: his odds of surviving the surgery, the odds of coming out of it in worse shape, how much more time it might buy him, and how long his recuperation might be afterward.[7]

In the end, however, what sealed the decision was whether he would still be able to enjoy a bowl of ice cream while watching a football game on TV after the surgery. If that seemed possible, life would be worth continuing. He had the surgery.

Before you get into trying to figure out which interventions you'd want to keep you alive, like heart resuscitation, a ventilator (breathing machine), dialysis, or IV fluids, start thinking about your *values* and the overall story of your life, Warshaw suggests.

Thomas offers the same message: When you're close to death, "a lot of things are happening to your body at the same time." Doctors, patients, and families can become so focused on treating failing organs that "they miss the big picture," she says.

You've already used your values to help you determine your meaning—or mission or purpose—for your life and job, and as a couple and family. Now, use that same strategy to help you estimate what you might want at the very end. Would you want every treatment that doctors could provide to avoid death a while longer, no matter how difficult your life becomes?

Or at some point, if further treatment isn't likely to allow you to enjoy your must-have experiences, would you be ready to meet your death? If so, what's your cutoff? What is your equivalent of ice cream and TV? What quality of life do you need to have in order to continue living? The answers to these questions reveal your values.

Once your wishes take shape, put them in a legal document called an advance healthcare directive. According to Thomas's organization, you don't need an attorney to fill out this form.[8] It offers a version on its Web site (coalitionccc.org), which is aimed at Californians but usable in other states. CaringInfo, a program from the National Hospice and Palliative Care Organization (NHPCO), also offers state-specific forms on its Web site (caringinfo.org).[9]

Another organization, called Five Wishes, offers an online document (go to agingwithdignity.org) for a small charge. It guides you through a variety of options that might be available at the end of life, like life support in a variety of scenarios; types of symptom relief or comforting measures; specific ways for people to interact with you; the location where you'd like to die (like hospital or home); and where you want your body to go (cremation? burial?).[10]

This document provides a useful way to think about your options, though at the time of this writing, in eight states you'll still need to fill out additional documentation to meet the legal requirements for an advance directive.[11]

Once you begin filling out your advance directive, you may find that your choices are simpler than you might expect, given the gravity of the situation. On the CaringInfo form for my state, some of the options essentially read:[12]

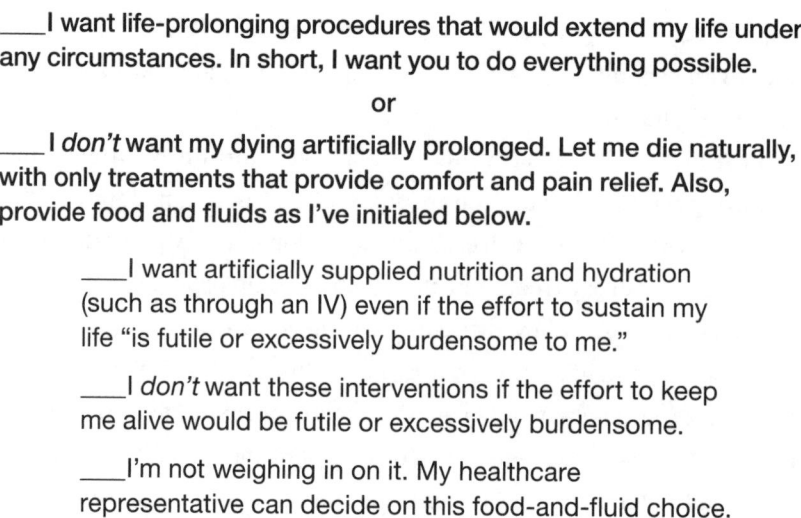

_____I want life-prolonging procedures that would extend my life under any circumstances. In short, I want you to do everything possible.

or

_____I *don't* want my dying artificially prolonged. Let me die naturally, with only treatments that provide comfort and pain relief. Also, provide food and fluids as I've initialed below.

> _____I want artificially supplied nutrition and hydration (such as through an IV) even if the effort to sustain my life "is futile or excessively burdensome to me."

> _____I *don't* want these interventions if the effort to keep me alive would be futile or excessively burdensome.

> _____I'm not weighing in on it. My healthcare representative can decide on this food-and-fluid choice.

You can also declare your wishes regarding organ donation. In addition, the document allows you to authorize someone to make healthcare decisions on your behalf, and it provides space for additional directions you'd like them to follow. This person may be referred by different titles depending on your location, such as an *agent, proxy,* or *advocate.* You may provide this person with *power of attorney* to make these decisions.

Once you've created this document, it's important that it remain available for the people who'll need it if you're in a life-threatening situation and can't speak. So make copies and distribute them to your agent who'll speak for you, as well as to your other close loved ones. Ask your doctor to put the form in your medical record, Thomas's organization advises.

Whatever you do, don't just lock one copy in your safe or bury it in a drawer. Tell the people around you what it says when you hold The Big Conversation. Ask them what they think about your wishes.

Step 3: Pick the Right Person to Represent You

Whenever he helps people choose a healthcare agent to speak on their behalf, Bud Hammes, PhD, asks them, "Can and will this person be able to make complex decisions in a stressful situation?" Roughly 20 percent of the time, "they look at me and smile and say no," he says.[13]

Dr. Hammes directs an end-of-life planning program at Gundersen Health System in La Crosse, Wisconsin. In all likelihood, the residents of La Crosse County do the most thorough end-of-life planning in the country, and possibly the world. Dr. Hammes says that 96 percent of adults who die in the county had an end-of-life care plan in their medical records, and their providers followed their preferences 99 percent of the time.

Make sure your healthcare agent—whether a spouse, adult child, sibling, or nonrelative—will be able and willing to advocate for your wishes when the time comes, he urges.

Are you considering someone who is unreliable in a crisis? Probably not your best choice. Do they have religious values regarding end-of-life situations that would hinder them from carrying out your wishes? Again, perhaps best to keep looking, he says. Ideally this person would live close enough to observe any changes in your health or quality of life in real time. But if your best choice is an adult child who lives 1,000 miles away, then that shouldn't preclude him from being your advocate, Dr. Hammes says.

Other important qualities, according to the American Bar Association, are that this person be an adult who:[14]

- You can trust with your life
- Can push for your wishes if a doctor or institution is "unresponsive" to requests
- Can handle conflicting opinions from family, friends, and healthcare providers
- *Isn't* a provider or administrator in a healthcare or residential facility that's currently serving you, or an employee or the spouse of an employee of your healthcare provider

Be sure this person is willing to accept the role's responsibilities and will continue to discuss your end-of-life wishes as they evolve over the coming years. The Coalition for Compassionate Care of California recommends you pick only *one* person to fill this role (joint advocates may disagree about how to interpret your wishes), but it is a good idea to select an alternate if the first choice is unavailable when necessary.[15]

Your advocate needs a copy of your advance directive, and you should have a plan in place for how they'll be notified if you're in a life-threatening situation that needs their involvement. Their contact information can go into your medical record as part of your advance directive. You may also want to carry a card in your wallet that names this person and provides contact information, Dr. Hammes says.

Step 4: Head Off Turmoil When Possible

Earlier in her career, Betty Kramer, PhD, was interviewing workers at a senior services agency. When she asked about challenges clients faced at the end of life, they repeatedly mentioned family conflict. She checked out a hospice and discovered that family turmoil commonly arose there, too.

When a loved one is dying, emotions tend to run high, she says. Families may be struggling to understand difficult medical concepts, cope with terrible news, bear their grief, and weigh the merits of options when none seem ideal. At these times, people don't necessarily display their best qualities.

However, if your family erupts in conflict when your death is close, it can have a negative impact on all of you, Dr. Kramer warns. Decisions may be delayed. Those wishes you expressed long ago might not be implemented. Conflicts can add to your loved ones' distress, and they could cause division among your family members that could take a long time to repair, if repair is even possible.

Commonly, turmoil arises from these sources, she says.

- Loved ones have different views on how sick the patient is or what kind of care they need. Often, one of them is a family member who has arrived in town from a faraway residence and who isn't as familiar with the patient's health status or wishes as the local contacts are. This "out-of-towner" phenomenon seems to occur all around the world, Dr. Hammes says.

- Participants have their own agendas. Perhaps they're jockeying for more of the estate, or they want to save money by withholding an expensive treatment or trip to a nursing home. Dr. Kramer shared the story of an adult daughter pleading with her dying father to wake up so she could borrow some cash.

- Family members with a medical or nursing degree may have their own ideas for the best course of action.

- The dying patient has a stigmatized or "avoidable" disease—like cirrhosis from drinking or emphysema from smoking—and families don't feel compelled to agree to more treatment.

- Or, the family simply can't accept the reality that their loved one is at the end. Again, the out-of-town relative may crave more conversations or experiences to help make up for the past distance or absence.

To help reduce the chances of deathbed conflict, start applying these strategies now.

Keep the lines of communication open. Be sure to express your end-of-life wishes and values to anyone who might show up expecting to be heard. Invite them to your inaugural Big Conversation. Keep them updated on any changes in your health, or whenever you have a shift in your thinking about the care you'd want at the end of your life, Dr. Kramer says.

You may have created legal documents expressing your wishes, but if a loved one first learns of them as you're dying, it's likely these will be perceived as just some writing on a piece of paper, Dr. Hammes says. It will be harder for this person to comprehend and honor the details you've provided than it would be if they had heard the same words coming directly from you much earlier and in a less emotional environment.

Examine old conflicts and the potential for new ones. Do any of your family members butt heads frequently or collide over the same recurring issues? Does a particular loved one often stir up conflict? Have old family crises gone unresolved, or have old hurts lingered unforgiven? Patterns of discord might predict future conflict, Dr. Kramer says.

Unrecognized fault lines may also start rumbling at the end of your life. Alliances and allegiances may shift within your family, particularly if it's a blend of stepparents and stepsiblings, she says.

Start examining these potential causes of conflict (and the others mentioned above). How could your family start conducting itself more peacefully? Would some of the strategies throughout this book—like practicing forgiveness, acceptance, and mindfulness, and holding family meetings to discuss shared values—be helpful? If you can anticipate conflict ("Oh yeah, I can see *this* individual raising *that* kind of fuss!"), could you start having conversations now that might keep it from happening?

Recruit help as needed. Sometimes families get stuck in a conflict that's so stubborn they need an outside professional, such as a mediator. You can already find mediators who specialize in healthcare and senior issues, and Dr. Kramer suspects that end-of-life disagreements will be a growing specialty for mediators in the future.

If your family ever needs to find consensus on an optimal solution, this professional may be able to play a valuable role. Ask your lawyer or your hospital for suggestions on finding a mediator in your area.

Step 5: Stay Flexible

Harriet Warshaw's mother fought breast cancer, throat cancer, colon cancer, and lung cancer over the years, and she decided near the end of her life that she didn't want more chemotherapy that a doctor was recommending. The family decided to meet to consider what their future held.

While they were together, Warshaw's mother heard her grandson Matt studying for his bar mitzvah, and she decided she wanted to live long enough to celebrate the ceremony with him. (That's an example of a value.) She returned to her oncologist, began chemo, and lived long enough to share this important occasion with Matt. Eventually, she died of emphysema. (*That's* an example of death not following one's expectations.)

The Conversation Project recommends that people revisit their end-of-life planning periodically, Warshaw says. Maybe you'll want to review it every 5 years, or even annually, if necessary, to see if your wishes have evolved or you want to recruit a new healthcare advocate. Other big changes that might prompt a review of end-of-life plans include:

- Getting married or divorced
- The death of a loved one
- Having children
- A significant change in your health

As a healthy 36-year-old, pulmonary and critical care specialist Lauren Van Scoy, MD, told me that she'd be willing to ask for aggressive medical interventions in an emergency to stay alive. But, "if I were 96, I would probably *not* be very aggressive in my care. Or if I weren't healthy, I might see it differently," she says.[16]

There's an easy way to learn more about the shifts in your values and wishes that might occur over the coming decades, Dr. Van Scoy says. Can you guess what it is? You've seen it before. Have you started doing it yet?

That's right: "Talk to an older person. Ask them, 'What would you have thought when you were 50, 70, or 90?'" she says. Did they once feel certain they'd want to stay alive at any cost, but their attitudes have changed? If so, why? Or did they encounter some reason to move in a *different* direction?

If your wishes change, remember to let others know. Hold another family conversation. Put your requests in legal-strength documents and circulate them to the people who need to have them. (It's wise to destroy your old versions and ask your loved ones to do the same.)

Try to get everyone on the same page now. Because if you don't, the people close to you may be unable or unwilling to meet there at the end of your life.

Research Finds Wishes Shift with Time, Circumstances

If you change your mind about your end-of-life wishes, you won't be alone.

In a 2013 study that reviewed earlier research, the authors found that the majority of people wished to die at home. However, roughly one-fifth of people with illnesses saw their preference change as their condition progressed.[17]

A 2016 study, which involved people hospitalized within the Kaiser Permanente Northern California system, found that it was more common for patients ages 85 and older to request that lifesaving treatments be limited (54 percent) compared to patients younger than 65 (3 percent).

These older patients were also six times more likely to change their wishes to ask for more limitations (in other words, to turn down more lifesaving treatments) than the under-65 crowd.[18]

LIVE WELL, DIE HAPPY EXERCISES
Chapter 11

1. Watch a documentary—or more than one—about the decisions that people face at the end of life. Good options include *Being Mortal,* produced for PBS and based on the Atul Gawande book of the same name; *Extremis,* a moving short that was filmed in an Oakland, California, hospital; and *Time of Death,* a Showtime series. All are available for streaming at the time of this writing.

2. Make a list of the values that might affect the type of medical interventions you'd want to keep you alive. Do you see life as a gift that you're obligated to extend for as long as possible? Do you take pride in being a fighter? Might you want to make a decision that causes the least distress to your family?

3. Think about the quality of life you would need in order to want to continue living, if you had a life-threatening medical condition. Would you be okay with not being able to walk? Think clearly? Communicate? Live on your own? People can find meaning and happiness despite a lot of adversity. What would you still need to be able to do in order to make life worth living?

4. After reading Chapter 12, complete a legally valid advance directive, including specifying your healthcare agent.

5. When you're finished with your advance directive, gather your loved ones for a conversation about your wishes, and be sure that everyone who needs a copy of your advance directive gets one.

Discussing End-of-Life Decisions with Your Healthcare Providers

When death seems imminent but you're determined to stay alive at any cost, a hospital is not a bad place to be.

"If the goal is to keep the patient alive in any state, we frequently can get a pulse back. We have a lot of medical interventions and medicines that help us do so. When other organs like the kidneys or lungs fail, we have machines that can replace them," says Lauren Van Scoy, MD, assistant professor of medicine and humanities at the Penn State Milton S. Hershey Medical Center in Hershey, Pennsylvania.[1]

Once the staff has determined to "code" a patient (in other words, resuscitate), the scene gets intense.

"The nurses shift the patient to their side and throw a backboard under them. That's so when they do chest compressions, it's against something hard instead of the soft bed. And then someone gets on the patient's chest, usually with their knees on the bed, and pushes really hard and really fast. Usually, two or three interns line up and rotate, because it takes so much energy you can only do it for 2 minutes at a time," she says.

This brings to mind a CrossFit workout.

"It really is! You sweat!" she says. "One doctor, usually the most senior, is usually at the foot of the bed directing the process. Someone's getting the IV, and someone's pulling the gown off the patient to attach the EKG leads, and someone's passing a needle. If the family is in the room, they're often upset and huddled in the corner watching. Sometimes families may feel skeptical that the team isn't going to do everything, which can cause tension. So watching the team work can be a good thing. Also, it can be informative for the family to see that this isn't just a 'tap, tap, tap' on the chest. It's serious stuff."

Discussing your end-of-life wishes with your family is one matter, with its own potential difficulties. But talking with your healthcare providers about this serious stuff may not be easy, either.

End of Life May Pose "Should I Stay or Should I Go Now?" Question

Many people enter the healthcare system near the end of their life. Out of a group of more than 4,100 seniors who died over a 14-year period, 51 percent visited an emergency room in the last month of their life, according to a study in *Health Affairs*. Of these, 77 percent were admitted to the hospital, and 68 percent of this group died there.[2]

Recent statistics have also shown that nearly 29 percent of people with cancer were admitted to an intensive care unit (ICU) in their final month, and one in five Americans in general receives care there near the end of life.[3, 4]

Generally speaking, if you or a person acting on your behalf (who's ideally backed up by your advance directive) *don't* specify otherwise, healthcare providers are obligated to keep you alive through medical interventions when your heart stops. That means getting oxygen into your lungs and keeping your heart beating, says Judy Thomas, JD, the CEO of the Coalition for Compassionate Care of California.[5]

Someday, you or your spokesperson might need to decide if prolonging your life is the right choice for you.

The providers you encounter at the end of your life aren't necessarily going to urge you to undergo aggressive treatments. When patients have a minimal chance of meaningful recovery, the doctors and nurses keeping them alive in these hospital rooms may wonder, "Why are we doing this? Are we really helping our patients?" Dr. Van Scoy says.

Ferdinando Mirarchi, DO, clinical assistant professor of emergency medicine at the University of Pittsburgh, echoed this sentiment. "What you hear in the media today is essentially that doctors are overutilizing resources and not letting people die, and that's not really the case," he says.

"Doctors get moral fatigue. It's *hard* to keep taking care of chronically ill patients when you're basically putting them through the same thing over and over with no benefit. Doctors like to make decisions so that if a treatment is beneficial, they'll continue it," he says. When a treatment is not expected to offer a benefit, they might advise against it.[6]

But ultimately, every case is different, so your healthcare providers need to know *your* values and goals in order to make decisions that are right for you. And often these days, they don't receive this information and must proceed without it.

"In general, across the population, it's pretty clear we end up doing things to people that they wouldn't necessarily say they want," says Malcolm Mattes, MD, assistant professor of radiation oncology at West Virginia University in Morgantown. "I think we put people through things toward the end of life because we don't ask them to think about their own mortality in advance. We don't ask them what's important to them."[7]

At the end of life, the best path to take isn't always obvious. But the questions you've answered throughout this book will help point you—or the person making decisions on your behalf—toward ideal options. Knowing how to speak with your healthcare providers can make it easier to acquire additional illumination. The following 10 ideas can make these conversations more productive.

Step 1: Discuss the Values That Can Shape the Rest of Your Story

One of the first papers that a medical journal accepted from Hunter Groninger, MD, was an essay about Samuel Beckett's play *Rockaby*. His take was that the work, which explores "how the elderly prepare for life's end in a death-denying culture," can teach healthcare providers "how we all must manage one day the . . . act of dying." A literature student before going to medical school, Dr. Groninger is now the director of palliative care at MedStar Washington Hospital Center in Washington, DC.[8]

Not surprisingly, he suggests that you give your story a central role in determining the best approach at the end of life. Often, a life-threatening health problem arrives like an unwelcome plot twist. "You can describe it as a broken narrative: 'This ended up with a different ending I don't like! I was going to be a husband and father of four kids, and this isn't how it worked out.' Or, 'I just retired last week and had all these things planned, and *this* week I was diagnosed with end-stage cancer.'"[9]

To understand how best to respond to such developments in your story, review the *meaning* you've made for your life. Remember that meaning helps give your life a coherent flow, like a thoughtfully written book or movie. You act according to consistent values, and over time your decisions accumulate to create a life that makes sense.

Also, think about the values that have driven your life thus far, and use them to inform any goals that you want to accomplish with your medical care, says Canadian critical care physician Simon Oczkowski, MD. That strategy is in direct contrast to a more common approach: finding out which treatments are available and picking one.[10]

"When we have end-of-life discussions, so often physicians are quick to talk about, 'Are we going to do dialysis? Mechanical ventilation? CPR?' I think we do our patients a great disservice when the focus is all about tests and treatments. I find the most rewarding processes at the end of life come when patients, families, and physicians have a rich discussion and bring their expertise to the table," he says.

"The patients and families are the people who are best able to decide what the goals of care are. What is a good enough quality of life? How much uncertainty can you tolerate around the outcome? How long are you willing to undergo tests or treatments to get there? Answering these questions requires talking about who you are, what is important to you, and what your previous life experiences have taught you about suffering and recovery. If everyone agrees on these decisions, you have this great plan going forward that brings together the best knowledge and expertise of everyone involved."

Step 2: Give Providers the Space to Talk

Sometimes, both patients and doctors are reluctant to start important discussions at the end of life. Be ready to show that you're okay with weighty conversations, even if they might lead to bad news or difficult decisions.

"It's hard to know when to say to a patient and family, 'I think things aren't going well. I think we should start thinking about what we want the rest of your time to look like.' That's a hard thing for a lot of clinicians to say," says Meredith MacMartin, MD, a palliative care doctor and assistant professor at Dartmouth's Geisel School of Medicine in Hanover, New Hampshire.[11]

"I think for patients and families, if they have the sense that 'Boy, things don't seem like they're going well,' it's okay to talk about it. If they feel that their physician is uncomfortable, it's okay to ask, 'How much longer do you think I have? What do you think my future holds for me?'"

Dr. MacMartin mentioned a *Washington Post* essay by prominent palliative care physician Diane Meier, MD. She wrote about the case of a patient who came to her office because, after years of successfully fighting lung cancer, she couldn't get her oncologist to discuss what they would do if the treatments stopped working.[12]

Eventually, her disease did worsen. The oncologist recommended an invasive approach to the patient—chemotherapy directly into her brain to treat a growth—but admitted to Dr. Meier on the phone that he didn't think it would help. "It seemed that giving more treatment was the only way the oncologist knew to express his care and commitment. To him, stopping treatment was akin to abandoning his patient," she wrote.

Sometimes, doctors are also concerned about distressing patients and their families during an already challenging time, Dr. Van Scoy says. "It's really the doctor's job to bring it up, but sometimes they're afraid of upsetting families. Because there are so many people who react badly if you talk about end of life, if you're the type of person who *does* want to talk about it, let your doctor know!"

"How Long Do I Have?" Isn't So Easy to Answer

If your doctor estimates how much time you have left, it's best to think of the number as an educated guess rather than a fact.

A 2013 review of earlier research in the *Journal of Supportive Oncology* found that physicians treating people with advanced cancer are correct when predicting their life expectancy only 20 to 60 percent of the time. Generally, they *over*estimate the amount of time patients have. In one study, doctors who knew their patients longer gave less accurate estimates (each year of familiarity raised the odds of an inaccurate prediction by 12 percent).[13]

In 2016, researchers asked cardiologists, oncologists, and internal medicine physicians to predict survival in three sample patients, one with Stage 4 lung cancer and two with heart failure. The doctors were more accurate in estimating survival for lung cancer (74 percent) than heart failure (48 percent).[14]

Your doctor's estimate can be important for guiding your next steps. But it's also a good idea to ask what you might do to improve your prognosis, and if there are any signs that could indicate whether you're likely to live for more (or less) time than has been predicted, said palliative care physician Ira Byock, MD, when speaking to an American Society of Clinical Oncology publication.[15]

"Although knowing your prognosis can be helpful for making important personal plans, it is just one of many factors to consider when you are striving to live fully with cancer," he added.

Step 3: Remember Your Shared Decision-Making Experience

When patients come into a situation knowing their values and providers bring information about treatment options and their expected results, they set the stage for shared decision making. (Remember that concept? It arose in Chapter 6 in relation to managing health problems earlier in life.)

When researchers recorded 51 end-of-life conversations between family members and physicians, they found that the more the family shared in decisions, the happier they were with the conversation. The discussion that determined how much they contributed to the decisions included: the treatment choices and their pros and cons; the likelihood that options would be successful; how well the family understood them; the patient's values and preferences; and the family's opinion on the decisions.[16]

To participate in a shared decision with your healthcare provider, think about the outcomes you hope to achieve. You'll want to discuss what you require from your life in order to continue it. (Must you be able to live independently? Communicate with loved ones? Live to see a granddaughter's wedding?)

But you also may need to drop some misconceptions at the shared decision-making table. According to the Institute of Medicine, people's input is sometimes overly influenced by:[17]

- Rare cases they once heard about in which the patient recovered
- The belief that their disease won't progress like the typical case (which goes back to the notion that "I shouldn't have to suffer from this because I'm somehow special")
- Someone else's experience that isn't relevant to the case at hand
- Incorrect ideas about how medicine works

You may also need to be flexible about ideas you've carried a long time about life-sustaining treatments. A blanket "I wouldn't ever want *that*" statement may not apply once you get there.

Consider the experience of one of Dr. Oczkowski's patients, who needed a pacemaker. He told her that during the procedure to implant the device, she would have a high chance of developing an irregular heartbeat that might require CPR. She told him, "I want to be walking my dog and hanging out with my family as long as possible. If that can't happen, I don't want to be on life support. I don't want CPR because of the risk of brain damage and long-term disability." But the CPR she pictured was based on an imagined situation in which her heart stopped and she collapsed, and her brain was deprived of oxygen for some time before paramedics arrived.

"The type of CPR we were talking about was 2 or 3 seconds while we put in the pacemaker wire," Dr. Oczkowski explained. "We'd be right there, the equipment would be right there, and her chances of brain damage were minimal. When the cardiologist and I explained that to her, she was okay."

If you come to a shared decision-making situation someday, be ready not only to speak but also to *listen*.

A Few Scenarios to Consider

In a 2016 study, researchers asked 180 people hospitalized with a serious illness (advanced cancer, congestive heart failure, or COPD) whether certain outcomes would be worse than dying.[18]

The majority felt that these scenarios would either be worse than death or neither better nor worse than death.

- Having bowel and bladder incontinence
- Requiring a breathing machine to live
- Inability to get out of bed
- Requiring a feeding tube to live
- Needing care all the time

On the other hand, more than half felt that the following situations would be *better* than dying:

- Needing a wheelchair
- Having moderate pain all the time
- Being at home all day
- Living in a nursing home

What's your opinion on these outcomes? If you're reasonably young and healthy, do you think your impression might be different if you were at the end of life? Spending more time around people who are elderly or extremely ill could give you a better understanding of what it's really like to live with these situations, in case you ever have to factor them into a decision.

Step 4: Try to Determine Whether You're Really at the End of Life

People don't always navigate the end-of-life process as planned, and Dr. Mirarchi is at the forefront of pointing out some of the cracks that patients can inadvertently fall into.

He urges patients and their advocates to get a clear understanding from their healthcare providers of where they stand.

- **Are they truly at the end of life?** Have they arrived at the very end of a terminal illness or sustained a catastrophic injury that is incurable or untreatable, and life-sustaining treatments (the ventilator, the dialysis, the CPR) will only delay an inevitable death from these causes?

- **Do they have a critical—but treatable—illness?** Or is this an emergency that's life-threatening, but potentially reversible? After treatment, which might require aggressive resuscitation and invasive procedures, could the patient go back out into the world with a satisfactory quality of life?

"Frankly, end-of-life care planning is getting the buzz, and so much stuff that gets lumped into what's called end-of-life care is really critical illness," he says. If your advance directive, along with all those conversations you had with your loved ones, were aimed at end-of-life but someday they become applied to a critical illness from which you might recover, you may not get the lifesaving treatment you'd really want, Dr. Mirarchi says.

Step 5: Ask about the Implications of Your Choice

Often, when doctors are trying to keep you alive in an urgent situation, their priority is *right now,* and they might not be too focused on your quality of life a few months down the road, Dr. Van Scoy says. But *you*—or your healthcare agent—should be.

If you agree to a particular life-sustaining intervention, will you need a year of rehabilitation afterward to regain physical functions? Will you need to move out of your house and into a nursing home? What quality of life can you expect? These are important questions to ask, she says.

Compare your medical providers' answers to your values and goals. Whether or not they match up should help determine your next move.

Step 6: Accept Ambiguity

When you can accept the present moment (page 90) and improve your tolerance of uncertainty (page 93), you may find yourself better able to navigate end-of-life situations. Sometimes life and death have just enough space between them to create ambiguity.

"One of the biggest difficulties when someone's getting sick and we're deciding, 'Are we going to put them on life support?' is the uncertainty of whether they'll get better," Dr. Oczkowski says.

"Lots of times patients will say, 'I don't want life support for a long time. But if it's something I can get better from, I do want it.' Then they get pneumonia, you put them on a ventilator, and there's a lot of gray area where it's unclear if they're going to get better," he says. "When I put someone to sleep and put in a breathing tube and put them on life support, once in a while I'm talking to the patient, they go to sleep and never wake up, and I'm the last person they ever see."

Making choices that match your values and goals may require reappraising your situation as it evolves, Dr. Oczkowski says. The best choice yesterday—or even hours ago—may not be the best choice now. And the best choice now may not be black and white.

Step 7: Ask More Than Just, "What Would You Do?"

It's common for patients to ask their doctors what choice they'd make for themselves or a relative in the same situation. It's a good question, Dr. Oczkowski says. But don't limit yourself to asking which option your doctor would choose; ask *how* she would come to that decision.

While her values, goals, and the outcomes she'd want from her choice will likely be different from yours, and thus not directly applicable to your case, the insight is valuable. The factors that your doctor would consider might provide helpful information, like the odds that an option would succeed or the risk that it might cause a harmful result.

Often, Doctors Wouldn't Want the Treatments They Provide at the End of Life

In an essay that went viral in 2011, physician Ken Murray, MD, reflected on the invasive, "futile" care that many seriously ill patients receive at the end of life.[19]

"The patient will get cut open, perforated with tubes, hooked up to machines, and assaulted with drugs. . . . What it buys is misery we would not inflict on a terrorist." Doctors, however, "don't die like the rest of us," he wrote.

"What's unusual about them is not how much treatment they get compared to most Americans, but how little. For all the time they spend fending off the deaths of others, they tend to be fairly serene when faced with death themselves. They know exactly what is going to happen, they know the choices, and they generally have access to any sort of medical care they could want. But they go gently."

A 2014 study from Stanford backs up this sentiment. More than 88 percent of doctors surveyed said they'd want to be "no code" at the end of life. Specifically, that meant, "I do not want my life to be prolonged if the likely risks and burdens of treatment would outweigh the expected benefits, or if I become unconscious and, to a realistic degree of medical certainty, I will not regain consciousness, or if I have an incurable and irreversible condition that will result in my death."[20]

The researchers noted that 80 percent of people say they don't want to be hospitalized and given high-powered treatments at the end of life, yet this is often what the modern healthcare system provides. "This study raises questions about why doctors provide care to their patients, which is very different from what they choose for themselves and also what seriously ill patients want," they concluded.

Step 8: Beware of Unintended Consequences

In the mid-1990s, Dr. Mirarchi was preparing to defibrillate a patient whose heartbeat was fluttering fast and out of control. (This is the "shout *clear* and shock with the paddles" maneuver you've seen on TV.)

"A nurse came in saying, 'Don't treat her, don't treat her. She has a living will,'" he says. But she didn't say what the living will said to do. An intern at the time, Dr. Mirarchi struggled to figure out the right move.

"Fortunately, a cardiologist happened to be in the unit and pushed me aside. He shocked the lady, and she lived and walked out of the hospital. Had he not been there, she would have died. She was maybe 50 years old at the time," he says.

Since then, the emergency physician has taken a strong position in the national conversation about advance directives, do not resuscitate (DNR) orders, and Physician Orders for Life-Sustaining Treatment (POLST) documents. "They are good documents that are very well intended, but they can have unintended consequences. The consequences are a safety risk to you as a patient. These documents can make you live longer, or they can make you live shorter, depending on who's utilizing or interpreting them," he says.

By "living shorter," he means dying earlier than you really envisioned, perhaps with some good life left in you.

dic·tio·nary

DNR (Do Not Resuscitate)

This is a medical order, typically written by a physician, that tells healthcare providers not to perform CPR if your heart stops beating or you stop breathing. Emergency physician Ferdinando Mirarchi, DO, recommends that you complete a DNR only if you have a terminal illness.

CPR often isn't a miracle cure, especially for people who are already very sick. In a study of more than 84,000 people who went into cardiac arrest (their heart stopped beating) in a hospital and had CPR, the number who were discharged alive from the hospital varied from 13.7 percent in 2000 to 22.4 percent in 2009. During that later year, 28 percent of these patients who left the hospital had a significant degree of brain-related disability.[21]

dic·tio·nary

POLST

This stands for Physician Orders for Life-Sustaining Treatment. Each state has its own version, and the name may vary somewhat, says Judy Thomas, JD, the CEO of the Coalition for Compassionate Care of California.[22]

This is a medical document your healthcare professional completes that puts your treatment wishes into easily understandable medical directions for others to use in an emergency. They're typically printed on blazingly pink paper that catches everyone's attention. (Picture a posterboard sign advertising a yard sale). After your healthcare provider fills out your form, you should keep it in a prominent place in your home, like on the front of your refrigerator. A few states also have an electronic registry to store individuals' POLST forms.

A POLST form is intended for people with an advanced disease, like heart disease or cancer, who are not expected to live more than a year, Thomas says. It's also intended to *supplement*—not replace—the advance directive you should have completed earlier.

Since 2008, Dr. Mirarchi and colleagues have published seven studies (at the time of this writing) in a series called TRIAD (The Realistic Interpretation of Advanced Directives). These surveys asked EMTs, paramedics, nurses, medical students, and doctors how to respond to sample scenarios in which patients had advance care planning documents. Across the studies, healthcare providers showed a considerable amount of confusion and misunderstanding about whether or not to perform lifesaving interventions.

One concern, Dr. Mirarchi says, is that some documents may contain multiple pages written by attorneys, which professionals in the medical environment must interpret correctly in a matter of moments. Also, a series of checked boxes that the patient may have filled out long ago might be difficult to apply to an unclear situation.

"I'm 46. If you found me dead, I would not want you to resuscitate me. If you find me in an unwitnessed cardiac arrest situation, there's no hope for recovery," he says. In other words, if his heart stops while he's alone, causing an unknown degree of brain injury until help arrives, he doesn't want medical intervention. "But if someone *sees* me having cardiac arrest, that's a different ball game. Then you need to come at me with a full-court press. We try to use these yes or no checkboxes, and sometimes the answer is in the middle or just, 'it depends.'"

Another issue that troubles him is that after you first make contact with a medical provider, perhaps a paramedic or admitting nurse at the ER, your wishes regarding resuscitation may or may not pass to the rest of your providers accurately, but once they're released into the open, they can be hard to alter, he says.

Bud Hammes, PhD, the administrator of the advance care planning program at Gundersen Health System in La Crosse, Wisconsin, sees some validity in these concerns. But to him, it's no different than any area of medicine in which we hope the providers are well trained in their jobs and performing at the top of their skills. "Whether it's about surgical training or oncology training, any time we have healthcare providers who are inadequately trained to carry out the work we expect them to do, it's a danger to patients."

Other voices have also been pointing out the potential for shortcomings in advance directives in recent years.

" . . . [O]ne of the most sobering facts is that no current policy or practice designed to improve care for millions of dying Americans is backed by a fraction of the evidence that the Food and Drug Administration would require to approve even a relatively innocuous drug," wrote University of Pennsylvania critical care physician Scott Halpern, MD, PhD, in the *New England Journal of Medicine* in 2015.[23]

POLST programs have an "absence of compelling evidence that they improve patient outcomes," he wrote. He also put The Conversation Project, Five Wishes, and the Gundersen Health System's Respecting Choices program into the "needs more evidence" category.

In short, you can't expect advance care planning documents to work perfectly in every case. They aren't a guarantee that every step will go as you specified or that the paramedic, nurse, or doctor you might encounter someday will locate and accurately apply your wishes in an emergency situation.

This is why you saw the warning in Chapter 1 that end-of-life care can be akin to childbirth: When the big moment comes, it may not match your expectations. (In the meantime, as with other areas in healthcare, the experts are trying to improve the process.)

Still, that's no excuse to skip advance care planning. Here are a few steps that you can take to increase the chances that any life-sustaining treatments match your wishes.

- Again, *make sure* to pick a healthcare advocate whom you'd trust to make the best decision when the options aren't black and white. Have regular conversations over time to maintain a shared understanding of your wishes.

Woman Appreciates Medicine's Gifts, But Recognizes Its Limits

In the early 1980s, Ide Mills's mother lived for 3 years with lung cancer. Mills is now nearly 6 years into her own fight against the disease, and her survival has depended on a variety of treatments, including therapy that was still in clinical trials.

"I was diagnosed with it at Stage 4, and I've been on therapy ever since: chemotherapy, targeted therapies, and radiation therapy, both stereotactic (precisely focused) and whole-brain," says the 59-year-old, who pivoted from a long career as an oncology social worker into healthcare marketing. She's now a consultant, focusing on patient education and advocacy.

"If you just hear about Stage 4 lung cancer, you'd say, 'Oh no, she must be at death's door!' When someone hears that I have brain metastases, they probably say, 'Her time is limited.' Which it is! But I don't know when it is. I'm probably feeling stronger and better than I have in years. I'm doing pretty well."

Because her cancer has a certain kind of mutation, Mills's doctors

- Tell your medical providers whether you have an advance directive, a DNR, and/or a POLST form. Have a conversation during which you (or your representative) clearly state what you do or do not want done in the current situation. When possible, don't make the medical providers try to interpret your documents without your input.

- Remember that just because you go on life-sustaining treatments, like a ventilator, you're not committed to staying on them indefinitely. You and your medical providers may decide to try one of these approaches on a trial basis—say, 48 to 72 hours—and discontinue it if it's not providing the results you want, Dr. Mirarchi says.

still have more drug options to direct against it, if necessary. Immunotherapy may offer more possibilities, too. Still, she's had conversations with her husband and her oncologist about how to determine when it's time to stop fighting the cancer.

"I'm going to trust my body to say it's really had it, and one more treatment isn't going to save my life with a quality of life that's meaningful," she says.

In the meantime, she's trying to approach her disease with humor. "We live in an apartment, and I worry, 'Where will everyone sit shiva after the funeral?' Maybe we should have bought a bigger apartment with a balcony." And she's setting her goals within a moderate timeline.

"Do I want to see my kids get married and have grandchildren? Absolutely. I think that I probably won't see a grandchild, but if that's what's gonna be, that's what's gonna be," she says, her voice growing choked with emotion. "I don't have a bucket list, but I want to make sure I've made a difference in life. Maybe that's why I'm trying to do more advocacy right now. It may be a small difference, but still a difference. I'm not here just to take—I want to give back."

Step 9: Manage Your Expectations

When your life is in jeopardy, it's okay to hope for a miracle, but in the meantime you need to make rational decisions based on outcomes that are likely to occur, Dr. Oczkowski urges.

Every day, people become rich from the lottery, but that's not a reason for us to sell our homes to buy lottery tickets instead of investing in a retirement fund, he notes. Similarly, pushing yourself to the extreme ends of medical science in hopes of a miracle may be a plan you should reconsider.

"Almost every patient whom I take care of in the ICU, when you ask their family, they're fighters. Very few are characterized as 'giver uppers.' By the time people need the ICU or these tests and treatments, that tells you there's a human will to survive and it's in action," he says. "That being said, not everyone can be a miracle. Then it wouldn't be a miracle."

At the end of your life, the healthcare system may continue to offer options. One more procedure you could try, and then maybe another procedure after that, and this is what keeps you occupied until you die.

But a different path may be available to you—one that may *look* like doing nothing but is actually its own deliberate choice.

Step 10: Know When to Shift Your Focus

"Recently, we saw a patient who said, 'My doctor said we've got to do radiation and chemotherapy right now. Here's the schedule.' But this schedule doesn't fit with me going to choir practice twice a week and church on weekends!" Dr. Groninger says.

He raises a question that too few patients ask at the end of life: "When doctors say, 'You can do therapy A, B, or C,' what if patients asked, 'What if I didn't do any of these? What would that be like?' You can keep going to the hospital, in and out every other week, or you choose *not* to do that. You can choose something different. That's how the hospice alternative is often painted," he says.

Hospice doesn't mean giving up. It doesn't mean doing *nothing*. It merely means you're turning your attention elsewhere during your remaining time rather than fighting for a cure that's no longer likely to arrive. It means shifting your priority to staying comfortable.

"We try to get it into the heads of the house staff where we work that you never say, 'We're withdrawing care,'" Dr. Groninger says. "You can always provide care, but in a different way. You might withdraw dialysis, but that doesn't mean you're stopping all interventions. For many people, going home is a very therapeutic intervention."

And perhaps someday, this might be where your story reaches its conclusion: at home.

LIVE WELL, DIE HAPPY EXERCISES
Chapter 12

Since this chapter's discussion goes hand in hand with Chapter 11, make sure you've completed that chapter's exercises. Proceed with completing a legally valid advance directive and starting an end-of-life conversation with the people close to you.

_____

_____

_____

_____

_____

_____

_____

_____

_____

CHAPTER 13

Making the Most of the End of Your Life

"Any good book has a beginning, a middle, and an end. In our society, when we've decided to ignore the end of life, it's like we've torn out great chapters from a book. The ending is usually what ties it all together and lets the meaning of it all become obvious," Karen Wyatt, MD, told me.

A retired Colorado physician, Dr. Wyatt spent much of her career as a hospice medical director, and now she consults and writes about end-of-life issues.[1]

Most people say they want their story to end in the place where much of it transpired: at home. A study that compiled research from around the world found that up to 70 percent of the general public—and up to 87 percent of patients, most with terminal illnesses—want to be at home when the end comes.[2]

However, not everyone who expresses an interest in dying at home still wants it when death is near. In some cases, it simply doesn't work out because a caregiver may be overwhelmed or uncomfortable with death in the home. Sometimes the level of necessary personal or medical care makes dying at home impractical.

Whether you someday die at home, in a hospital, or in a nursing home, a pair of related strategies mentioned at the beginning of the book, palliative care and hospice, can help you put the finishing touches on your life story in a more comfortable manner.

How you proceed through your final months, weeks, and days truly matters. The care you receive for any physical discomfort will make a difference in how well you die, but so will the support you find for your emotional and spiritual well-being.

At the end of your life, how much time you have may matter less than *what you do with it*. And how "good" your death is will likely not be solely your concern. It can also affect how the people close to you cope with their loss after you're gone.

We're nearing the final pages of this book. As you were forewarned, it ends in death. Someday you'll arrive at your own final page: the Point B that finishes the line beginning with the present moment.

Until your death arrives, you can author a life that's overflowing with purpose and joy. This requires paying attention to the present moment, making deliberate choices, and embracing change. In your final days, this approach can also inspire a satisfying conclusion that ties up your loose ends and allows you to realize, "Yeah, *that's* what it was all about."

Here are some options to consider for how your last chapters might read.

Increase Your Comfort While You Hope for a Cure

If you develop a life-limiting disease such as cancer, heart disease, chronic lung disease, or stroke, at some point you might benefit from palliative care. Misunderstandings about this option keep a lot of people from discovering its benefits, so now is a good time to dispel some incorrect notions in case you need it someday.

The goal of palliative care is to "[mask] the symptoms of disease to improve the quality of life regardless of how much time remains," according to a recent article in *Critical Care Nursing Clinics of North America.* The name comes from *palliere,* the Latin word for "covering up with a garment." Palliative care can go beyond treating just your physical symptoms. It's also concerned with meeting your psychological, spiritual, and other needs.[3]

Palliative care is not intended to alter the underlying disease process. The purpose isn't to cure you, but to reduce the impact of how a disease is making you feel. Perhaps that's why there's a widespread perception among the public, and even some healthcare providers, that palliative care is just for people who are at the end of life.

In reality, it isn't.

Palliative care is also for people who do have a disease that will likely limit their lives, but who aren't at a terminal stage; people who are seriously ill now but may recover; and those who are receiving treatments to alter the course of a disease, but who also need better symptom relief.[4]

Research has found that this "palliative care is end-of-life care" misperception creates a substantial barrier that keeps patients from enjoying its benefits earlier. You might carry a more accurate view of this field of medicine by calling it *supportive care.* In one study, oncologists and other providers said they thought this term would feel less distressing and more hopeful to patients and families.[5]

In another study, set in the University of Texas M. D. Anderson Cancer Center, more patients had a first consultation visit with palliative care providers after their specialty had a name change to "supportive care." Patients also were referred to the service more quickly after they registered in the hospital or were diagnosed with advanced cancer.[6]

In some cases, palliative care options may seem as sophisticated as treatments intended to cure a disease. To manage pain, to use one common symptom as an example, a range of medications are available, including high-powered opioids. But in severe cases, palliative care might mean implanted tubes to drain accumulated fluid from within your abdomen or around your lungs, or an electronic device that delivers pain-relieving impulses through wires near your spinal cord.[7]

Palliative Care May Provide an Unexpected Benefit

In some cases, palliative care might improve not just the quality, but also the *quantity* of people's lives. In a 2010 study from the *New England Journal of Medicine,* doctors provided patients with recently diagnosed metastatic lung cancer with either standard care or standard care combined with early palliative care.[8]

People in the palliative care group reported fewer depression symptoms and a better quality of life. Also, though fewer of them had aggressive care at the end of life, they lived 2½ months longer than the group that didn't receive palliative care. (Their median survival was 11.6 months, compared to 8.9 months in the nonpalliative care group.)

Even low doses of radiation can be used for palliative purposes in people with late-stage cancer, says West Virginia University oncologist Malcolm Mattes, MD. If the cancer is growing within a bone, radiation may kill enough cells to relieve pain in the area. It may also reduce bleeding; shrink a tumor that's pressing painfully on a nearby structure; and treat neurological symptoms if cancer has spread to the brain or spinal cord.[9]

"When I think about patients who are kind of a slam-dunk for getting involved in palliative care early, it includes anybody with an incurable cancer, regardless of what their overall prognosis is," says palliative care physician Meredith MacMartin, MD, of Dartmouth's Geisel School of Medicine. "Anyone who has a diagnosis of metastatic or incurable cancer should at least have an intake visit with palliative care. They may not need to see them regularly at first if they're doing well, but I think establishing that relationship early is really helpful."[10]

People with cancer tend to be "ahead of the curve in terms of getting access to palliative care, but a lot of illnesses are still underserved," she says. She also recommends having an initial conversation with a palliative care provider if you have any other chronic, progressive, or advanced illness that's currently affecting your quality of life or will likely reduce the length of your life. Good examples of these include Parkinson's disease and ALS.

Another disease that can benefit from palliative care is heart failure, which affects nearly 6 million American adults.[11] Since the challenges associated with heart failure tend to fluctuate, with good stretches interspersed with worsening symptoms, it can be harder to know when to incorporate palliative care, Dr. MacMartin says. Fortunately, experts have issued guidance.

In a 2013 guideline for managing heart failure, the American College of Cardiology Foundation and the American Heart Association suggested palliative care and hospice as possible options for people with Stage D heart failure. (This is the final stage.)[12] And in 2016, cardiologist Jeffrey Teuteberg, MD, and palliative care specialist Winifred Teuteberg, MD, recommended on the American College of Cardiology Web site that people with heart failure see a palliative care provider if they're having:[13]

- Symptoms of NYHA Class III or IV heart failure, including fatigue, heart palpitations, and trouble breathing even with minor physical activity; discomfort during any physical activity; and heart failure symptoms at rest[14]

- Frequent hospital admissions for heart failure

- Repeated shocks from an implantable cardioverter defibrillator (a device that can jolt an abnormal heartbeat back into rhythm)[15]

- Chronic angina (chest pain)

- Anxiety or depression that reduces one's quality of life or ability to manage one's condition

- Certain treatment milestones, like receiving a heart transplant or a mechanical device that helps the heart pump blood

Another Sign for Palliative Care

Here's another benchmark that some experts say should prompt you to contact a palliative care provider: if your doctor would not be surprised if you were to die in the next 12 months. If you ever suspect that you would benefit from palliative care, ask your healthcare provider if it might be right for you.[16]

A 2016 study from the University of California, San Francisco, compared patients who were referred to palliative care early (more than 90 days before dying of cancer) with those who were referred late (fewer than 90 days before dying). Those who received palliative care earlier were less likely to go to the emergency room (34 percent versus 54 percent) and *much* less likely to be admitted to the ICU (5 percent versus 20 percent).[17]

If your goal someday is to spend as much of your limited time in comfort—and out of a hospital room—palliative care may support your cause.

Seek Greater Peace of Mind (and Body) at the End

At the end of life, hospice care often goes hand in hand with palliative care. In fact, you could say that hospice is a specific approach to delivering palliative care.

One way they're different is that hospice care is for people who truly are at the end of life. To be eligible—or at least for Medicare to pay for it—you must have a terminal illness expected to end your life within 6 months if it runs its normal course. Hospice care is intended to keep you comfortable and enhance your quality of life but not to cure the disease that threatens your life.[18, 19, 20]

Hospice isn't so much a place as it is a *concept*. You may receive hospice services in your own home, a nursing home, a freestanding hospice facility, or a hospital. A team of personnel provides care and typically includes one or more hospice physicians, nurses, social workers, chaplains, and volunteers, with assistance from your own doctor if necessary. You can call the hospice provider for emergency hospice care 24 hours a day as needed. Hospice may also provide bereavement support for your surviving loved ones. [21, 22]

As with palliative care, people frequently don't enroll in hospice early enough to derive its full benefits. Some experts feel that people at the end of life need at least 2 to 3 months to get the most value from participating in hospice. But in 2014, the median length that people used it was 17 days, according to the National Hospice and Palliative Care Organization. More than 35 percent used it for fewer than 7 days.[23, 24]

"Often if your doctor says, 'We should talk about hospice,' it should have been brought up a while ago," says Washington, DC, palliative care doctor Hunter Groninger, MD. He acknowledges that for many people, it's difficult to change course from an "I'm still going to beat this" mind-set that required a significant investment of their time, money, determination, and support.[25]

"There's a problem with its setup that you do one strategy up to a certain point, then quickly shift gears and do a different strategy. Life doesn't work that way: 'Monday I'm going for a cure, but if I get bad news, then Tuesday I'm going for hospice.' There's nothing magical about Monday to Tuesday. In reality, these transitions should take place over time," Dr. Groninger says.

Some experts now encourage clinicians to have these conversations in a more effective and timely manner. One leader in this field is author and surgeon Atul Gawande, MD. An organization he founded, Ariadne Labs, has developed a conversation guide that walks healthcare providers through the types of questions you've been learning to answer, covering:

- What your goals would be if your condition grows worse
- The abilities that are so important to you that you couldn't picture living without them

- How much treatment you'd be willing to tolerate if it offered the chance of more time

It also prompts your healthcare provider to ask you what you currently know about your health and how much you *want* to know about changes that might be coming.[26]

Dr. Gawande's colleague, Susan Block, MD, a fellow Harvard professor, has offered physicians guidance on the "triggers" that suggest it's time for an end-of-life conversation. These include the diagnosis of certain particularly serious diseases, like pancreatic cancer or glioblastoma (a type of brain cancer), or the need for certain therapies, like ongoing oxygen for chronic obstructive pulmonary disease (COPD).[27]

When we spoke, Dr. Groninger discussed a pilot endeavor that his hospital was testing for patients in its advanced heart failure program. Even though the doctors may be considering treatments that might improve their health, "when patients are referred to this program, they're almost always hospice eligible," he says. That is to say, their heart failure could be fatal in 6 months if the treatments aren't effective.

"We try to normalize the word *hospice* early. We tell them, 'There are lots of things we can do. Maybe you'll get drugs that will help your heart, or maybe a device or a transplant. And if your heart failure progresses, we'll be doing more supportive care,'" Dr. Groninger says. (You recognize that term, don't you? It's another name for palliative care.) "'At some point, we'll talk about this thing called hospice. We're not referring you today. We're just letting you know that it's in the spectrum of what typically happens in heart failure,'" he says.

"Anecdotally, we know that patients down the road, whether you do it 6 months or 5 years later, say, 'Oh yeah, you guys mentioned this.' They're not necessarily happy to be in that situation, but this is not news. It may help prevent some of the distress that comes with these conversations."

The Conversation Project, which I've mentioned several times throughout this book, also recommends a question to ask your healthcare provider that might bring hospice and palliative care into your discussion sooner: "Can you tell me what I can expect from this illness? What is my life likely to look like 6 months from now, 1 year from now, and 5 years from now?"[28]

If it's not likely to go beyond 6 months, the rest of your life may look like an opportunity to tie things up in a meaningful way.

Tap Into Life's Riches until the End

Again and again, people who bear witness at the ends of others' lives have spoken to me about the possibilities you may find during this period if you're open to them.

"People who are dying are still very much alive. They may be extremely weak, in pain, confused, and in and out of consciousness. The way they feel may be completely different from anything they have ever experienced so far in their lives, but they are still as alive. It's just a very different life," hospice chaplain Kerry Egan says.[29]

Palliative care specialist Dr. MacMartin voices a similar sentiment. "Being open to the possibility of growth even in the setting of serious illness is what I hope everyone is able to do. I've seen a lot of patients experience tremendous personal growth even toward the end of life."[30]

Someday, you might find that hospice care provides you with more resources to devote toward meaningful activities, Dr. Wyatt says.

"I think our medical process, when it's attempting to cure an illness, is all-consuming. All the focus for patients is on the regimen they're going through," she told me. "When people enter hospice, they stop trying to cure the physical body, and that's a huge mind-set shift. They stop fighting every single day to get treatments in a desperate attempt to keep the body alive. When they leave that aside and enter into hospice, they're wide open in terms of time and energy during the day, and space to consider other things."

If you still want to apologize for errors and offer forgiveness to others, you can find time here to check those items off your list, Dr. Wyatt says. You may also notice a newfound interest in appreciating the beauty of a sunset, a flower garden, and "all the little treasures of life you may have neglected in the past." (Hopefully you're already becoming more mindful of such fleeting splendor.)

"Almost everybody spends some time going back over, 'Here's what I've done with my life, here's what I would have done differently, here are my accomplishments, here are the things I'm proud of and the people I care about, and they're here with me.' It can make that death experience really a grand finale of maybe weeks and months of putting it all together," Oregon hospice nurse Amy Getter, MS, RN, says.[31]

Of course, you can still do these things at the end of life even if you aren't enrolled in hospice. But if you are, a social worker or chaplain on the team can help guide you through these sorts of issues.

Social workers play many roles throughout palliative care and hospice for patients and their families, like offering counseling and advice on coping with challenges, advocating for your needs, and mediating family conflicts, according to the National Association of Social Workers.[32]

Egan feels that the chaplain's role is to "help people look back on their life and make meaning and sense of all of it," she says. "Almost everybody who meets with a chaplain works on these questions of, 'What is it I believe that my life meant and means? In the last few months I have, who do I still want to become?' We're always becoming who we are up until the day we die. You change and grow until the moment you cease to be."

By the way, this is one of the benefits that people might not get to experience when they come to hospice just before they die. Egan has heard of patients dying during their admission appointment, before they even complete their paperwork.

For some, this journey to finding meaning involves their faith tradition. But even if you aren't particularly spiritual or religious, meeting with a chaplain may still have value, she says. You might discuss nonreligious sources of meaning you've experienced in your life, like work and family, and find language from songs and poetry to express your feelings.

The end of your life does not have to be a grim and bleak time for you and your family. Even after decades of living in the presence of death, Dr. Wyatt remains fascinated by the discoveries that reveal themselves during this time.

"For me, it feels really uplifting in some ways, just to see the tremendous beauty of the human spirit. I've seen so many patients who've had the opportunity to grow and reconcile with family members, or recognize, 'Boy, I would have done that differently' and come to peace with that, or to reconcile with their faith, or do some work on their legacy," she says.

"I think people are really magnificent. I've seen people who've had challenging lives and horrible medical circumstances, and for those people to still be so kind, and to share stories and laugh with me, speaks to the resiliency of the human spirit."

This Is How a Life Ends

Each person's death follows a course that's as individual as his or her fingerprints. But in general, people often encounter a similar set of symptoms at the end of life, according to the Institute of Medicine.[33]

Pain. Physical pain can also cause psychological distress and depression. Conversely, "sometimes when physical pain is out of control, it can be related to emotional or spiritual concerns," Dr. Wyatt says.

Reduced appetite and loss of muscle mass. Lack of interest in eating, and the related physical wasting, is especially common with dementia and end-stage cancer.

Weakness and fatigue. These symptoms may be due to a disease, its treatment, or a loss of appetite. Weakness and lack of energy can cause other problems, such as limited mobility or falls that lead to injury.

Trouble swallowing. Eating, drinking, and taking medications can become more difficult as the ability to swallow worsens.

Shortness of breath. This symptom can further limit physical activities near the end of life.

Digestive issues. Nausea, vomiting, and incontinence are common sources of distress for people who are dying, and they can create additional challenges for their caregivers.

Mental and emotional changes. People may develop confusion near the end of life, and that may hamper their ability to care for themselves and communicate with healthcare providers and caregivers. They may also feel anxious and depressed.

As death draws near, you might begin to turn away from outside distractions like television, directing your thoughts inward, according to the National Hospice and Palliative Care Organization. Or you may feel like taking care of unfinished business, talking about your life in review with a loved one, and passing along final information that your family needs to know.[34]

In your last few days, you might eat and drink little. You may glimpse or have conversations with loved ones who have died before you. Your thoughts might turn toward needing to buy tickets and pack for a trip that will take you somewhere far away. You may sleep more and more. While you might remain conscious and able to communicate, for many people this becomes no longer possible.

At the very end, your hands and feet may grow cool, and your breathing ragged and irregular. The space between breaths might stretch out longer and longer, and eventually the next one never comes.

And just like that, you're no longer here.

LIVE WELL, DIE HAPPY EXERCISES
Chapter 13

1. Check out Mary Oliver's poem "The Summer Day." More than one patient has mentioned it to chaplain Kerry Egan, and it's easily found online. It ends with a question that all of us should ask ourselves regularly.

_____

_____

_____

_____

_____

_____

_____

_____

2. Pick a meaningful activity that reliably provides a sense of deep happiness, and go do it! Someday you won't be alive, but right now you are. So celebrate this moment like the gift that it is!

_____

_____

_____

_____

_____

_____

_____

_____

_____

CHAPTER 14

Planning a Meaningful Funeral or Memorial

The bagpiper had finished bagpiping, and the interpretive dancer had concluded her interpretive dancing. Five o'clock had arrived, and this was the time of day when the 92-year-old guest of honor, Mary, traditionally enjoyed her cocktail.

So the event's organizer, Gail Rubin, brought the gathering to a close.

She alerted the crowd, "It's time for cocktails!" and passed out commemorative cocktail napkins. The guest of honor didn't receive one, however, since this was her memorial service. She'd planned it months before, while she was in hospice care for COPD.[1]

"At the end of it, people were saying, 'That was the perfect way to celebrate Mary's life.' That's what a good memorial service or funeral will do," says Rubin, an Albuquerque funeral celebrant and author of *Kicking the Bucket List* and *A Good Goodbye: Funeral Planning for Those Who Don't Plan to Die*.

"I've heard people say, 'When I die, don't have a funeral for me.' But we need to go to the trouble of having a memorial service or funeral because we love that person, and we need to say goodbye to them in a ritual, ceremonial way," Rubin says.

"Grief never goes away—it just changes form. A funeral or memorial service helps people process their grief. If they don't have this public recognition, it's like the person just disappeared or dropped off the face of the planet."

dic•tio•nary

Funeral celebrant

A funeral celebrant helps plan and lead funeral or memorial services that tend to be nonreligious in nature. Bonus definition: At a funeral, the body is present. At a memorial service, it's not, though cremated remains may be present.

By planning ahead, you can create a service that both commemorates your life in the manner in which you lived and provides a meaningful epilogue for your loved ones to remember as they close the book on your life—and begin a new chapter of their own.

Thinking about the funeral or memorial you'd like to have requires you to acknowledge that you'll be dead at that point, which might be even more challenging than doing the end-of-life planning that recognizes that you'll someday be dying.

But as Rubin says (often enough that it's her catchphrase), "Talking about sex won't make you pregnant, and talking about funerals won't make you dead."

As with End-of-Life Choices, Our Death-Related Customs Are Changing

In a fascinating 2010 paper from the journal *Omega,* Burden Lundgren, PhD, RN, and Clare Houseman, PhD, RN, of Old Dominion University in Norfolk, Virginia, tied together the historical shifts in the nation's end-of-life medical care and its funeral practices.[2]

As you learned in Chapter 1, death struck the populace early and often in the 1800s. Infectious diseases were rampant. Death was highly visible and unsurprising; the authors note that some parents saved wine at their children's births to be used for either their children's weddings or funerals.

Handling the dead was a community affair. Friends and neighbors helped the bereaved family build the coffin, dig the hole, wash and dress the body, and carry it from the home to bury it.

You already know how the rise of modern medicine helped change our views on death. It became largely segregated among the elderly. It often occurred far away in a hospital, overseen by well-trained professionals. As a result, death became less visible and more surprising.

A similar shift happened with the funeral process, these authors write. Funeral directing became a profession, and it assumed responsibility for the care and handling of the dead. Preparing the body meant embalming it with chemicals and masking it with makeup. "As one funeral director stated, the body should be laid out 'so that there will be as little suggestion of death as possible.'"

Cemeteries also moved from city centers to the rural outskirts, taking them out of sight unless visitors made a special trip.

But American attitudes toward death and dying are evolving. Interest is growing in medical options at the end of life that may not have been popular or available for your parents and grandparents, such as hospice care that may help improve your chances of dying at home, if that's your wish.

Similarly, our funeral and memorial customs are becoming more flexible, says Josh Slocum, executive director of the Funeral Consumers Alliance and coauthor of *Final Rights: Reclaiming the American Way of Death*.[3]

In recent years, "I think we've lost a lot of the healing power of funerals because we've turned over the grieving process entirely to a third-party commercial sector. We no longer see ourselves as able to meaningfully participate in creating the funeral. We see ourselves as customers and spectators who pay for it to be put on before us," he says.

The first time he saw a dead body was at age 16 at his grandmother's funeral, which he found "unpleasant and artificial." He more fondly remembers the gathering at his aunt's house afterward, which attracted 70 family members.

"The adults were out in the living room drinking a toast to Grandma with her favorite drink, the dreadful sloe gin fizz, and telling stories. I remember cooking, telling stories about Grandma, crying and laughing at the same time, and just being there with family. That's what was important to me and felt like a community rebuilding, rather than the time we spent on formality."

Some recent cultural shifts—like the rising popularity of cremation—may be due to the cost of a traditional funeral. According to the National Funeral Directors Association, the median cost for an adult funeral with viewing and burial in 2014 was $8,500. Given the range in price for caskets, as well as additional charges for items like flowers and a headstone, the cost can go much higher.[4] A cremation could cost as little as a quarter of that amount.

For families scattered across great distances, simpler and less time-sensitive customs like cremation with a memorial service at a later date may also be more convenient.

Several organizations, including Slocum's, advocate for greater acceptance of at-home funeral rituals. If a loved one dies at home, in general you can legally keep the body there for at least 24 hours, according to the National Home Funeral Alliance. (Setting the home's temperature at 65°F helps keep things pleasant, Slocum says.)[5]

After that, state laws vary, and some call for the body to be embalmed or refrigerated. Some states also require families to hire a funeral director to handle certain tasks, such as removing the body, filing a death certificate, or supervising the disposition of the body.

Keeping a body in the home for visitors to say their goodbyes in an intimate setting has a long precedent, Slocum says. "We have a short memory—a lot of people have never heard of the concept of an undertaker-free funeral. But it's not a weird thing, and it's what most of humanity did before the last quarter of the 19th century."

These rituals aren't for everyone, but if they're what *you* want after you die—and that choice works for your family members—such options may provide some comfort during their bereavement.

Even though you'll be the center of attention at your funeral or memorial, make sure that you plan ahead so it provides your loved ones with a chance to have a meaningful goodbye.

Though the Service Focuses on You, It's for Your Loved Ones' Benefit

After Teddy Roosevelt's socialite daughter died insisting that she have no type of service, a friend was said to say, "I think it was a great mistake . . . it was hard on everybody. . . . Maybe she did not want people to say pompous things about her. But I think when someone is not given a farewell, you have a terribly uneasy feeling of their spirit hovering. It is as if a piece of music stopped before the final chord."[6]

In his book *Do Funerals Matter?* Baylor University grief expert William Hoy, DMin, writes that "humans have an undeniable need to make sense of death; funeral rituals are created by social groups as potential scripts to achieve this end." These rituals generally begin shortly after the death, "likely as a remedy to the chaos of early grief."[7]

As he notes, psychologist and prominent death researcher Therese Rando, PhD, says that funerals are "vital" for the process of grieving and mourning. Not only do they acknowledge that a community member has died, but these rituals also:

- Provide support to the survivors
- Encourage the bereaved to participate in structured activities at a time when they may feel adrift
- Recognize loved ones' loss
- Help the bereaved develop new relationships with the deceased and their living connections

In many cases, people don't do much to plan their ceremonies ahead of time. On the occasions when they do contribute, it's often to prepay for the service and to specify to their families what the service should include, Slocum says.

While you do earn kudos for planning ahead, sometimes advance work can actually make the ceremonies around your death *more* complicated. People may die while they're traveling, or when they're living in a nursing home that's far from the funeral home, throwing a wrench into their prepaid plans, he says. Or, if they die 20 years after they prepay for a service, few may still be alive and mobile enough to come to a lengthy visitation except for family, who may prefer to create their own gathering.

"There's lots of encouragement out there to get people to *tell* their children what their last wishes are. I think you should be *asking* your children what will be meaningful to them. Instead of looking at this as, 'I will lay down dictates that you're obliged by moral law to follow,' you ought to be saying, 'Loved ones, what will help you when I go? What will feel meaningful to you? You'll be the ones who are still around with a conscious mind. I won't,'" Slocum says.

You can find many ways to honor your life while providing meaning for your loved ones. The older woman whose memorial Rubin led emphasized one of her passions—cocktails—but made room for family participation. The bagpiper was a nephew, and the interpretive dancer was a granddaughter.

Thinking outside the box, so to speak, perhaps you could have a religious funeral ceremony, with a more informal memorial later at the bowling alley you frequent. Multiple rituals to commemorate your different facets are definitely an option, according to Dr. Hoy.

In his book, he shares a funeral director's story of a conservative-seeming lawyer who listened to the Grateful Dead on the weekends. After his death, his parents wanted him laid out in a suit, and his teenagers pushed for jeans and a Jerry Garcia tie. They compromised, and the man appeared in his suit for the visitation and his casual wear for the funeral.

Your funeral or memorial is one of those times when the elements of living well and dying happy are especially connected. Advance planning can help you create an event with the necessary purpose and meaning. Your send-off can tie together multiple elements of the life you lived: your family; your faith; your career and personal mission; and your ways of finding happiness. It can also help the ones you leave behind start their grieving process in a supportive environment.

This ritual marks a momentous occasion when you come to a fork in the road . . . and take several branches at once.

The legacy you created over your lifetime continues forward among the living, made from the stories you told, the wisdom you shared, and the actions you took that rippled outward. As the people who cared about you come together, they can start celebrating that legacy.

Perhaps your spirit, soul, spark, inner light—or whatever name you have for it, if you have one—goes off to its own destination.

Meanwhile, the body you occupied ventures off to a quieter realm—perhaps into the ground, into the sea, or into an urn.

But if you were to ask the ancient Stoics, that wasn't the most important part of you, anyway.

LIVE WELL, DIE HAPPY EXERCISES
Chapter 14

1. Give thought to whether you would want a conventional funeral, with the embalming, the visitation, the casket, and the procession to the cemetery, or something less traditional. Are your choices based on just your preferences, or does your family have some input? Or are you just doing what you think your peers and community would expect? _____

_____

_____

_____

2. Figure out who will pay for your service and, if applicable, cemetery plot. If you've already prepaid, review what you've requested, and evaluate whether your choices would still meet your survivors' needs. What will happen if you're far away when you die? What happens if the service you paid for isn't what your loved ones really want? If you haven't paid, who will pick up the tab—perhaps your spouse or your estate? Make sure enough funds are available to cover the cost so your kids don't have an unpleasant surprise or a difficult decision. _____

_____

_____

_____

3. What are some of your interests and passions you'd want celebrated at your funeral or memorial? Have a conversation with your friends and loved ones to express your wishes. _____

_____

_____

_____

4. What needs would your loved ones have from your funeral or memorial? How can you incorporate factors that they would find meaningful during their grief?

_____

_____

_____

_____

CHAPTER 15

A Quick Recap to Guide Your Next Steps

Whatever your future holds, its details are a mystery. But this much is known: You were given the amazing gift of time on Earth, which is truly a once-in-a-lifetime opportunity. You've also had the freedom to use this time to the best of your abilities. In fact, you still do.

So what are you going to do with it? How are you going to get the most value from your life that remains? Will you give more than you take? Will you impact others' lives in a positive way? Will you pursue a purpose? Will you leave the campsite cleaner than you found it?

These answers will not just affect the quality of your life, but also the legacy that outlives you, which will be built from the stories you tell, the deeds you do, the wisdom you pass down, the lives you touch, and the memories you leave for others.

Given what you've learned, are you ready today to live well?

Someday, will you be able to die happy? The choice is yours.

I've collected some of the highlights of the previous 229 pages into sort of a timetable. Revisit this chapter from time to time to make sure you're covering all the *Live Well, Die Happy* necessities in a timely manner.

Things to Do *at Least* Once in Your Life

- Find your meaning! This requires thinking about your strengths; settling on at least one value you'd like to improve in the world; and writing a mission statement. Remember—your meaning involves having a sense of purpose that connects to your family, your work, and your leisure time.

- Make your job a calling! This requires assessing your values, strengths, and personality; figuring out the work tasks you especially enjoy; and asking your boss how you can focus more on the tasks you like that fit well with these factors. Whenever you change employment, try to find a new job that feels like a calling— or try to reshape the new job so it fits this need.

- Create a legally valid will.

- Make sure your life is sufficiently insured for any loved ones who will need financial support when you're gone.

- Record the stories of the heirlooms you'll leave behind. Do it via video, longhand on paper, with photos, or online. But leave these stories where your loved ones can find them.

- Create an ethical will. Again, use the format of your choice, but leave it where your loved ones can find it. (You may even want to share it while you're alive.)

- Forgive anyone who's harmed you, if you're still bearing a grudge or wishing for revenge.

- Spend time with someone who's dying.

- Create an advance directive that specifies the type of medical treatment you would want if your life were in jeopardy due to illness or injury.

- Choose someone to represent your healthcare wishes in the event that you can't speak for yourself.

- Have a conversation to discuss your end-of-life wishes with those close to you.

- Develop a general sense of what a "good death" looks like to you.

- Discuss your funeral or memorial wishes with your loved ones, and seek their input, too.

Things to Do *at Least* Every Few Years or When You Undergo a Major Life Change

- Think about the values that make your life worth living.

- Evaluate whether the person you've chosen to be your healthcare advocate/agent/proxy is still the best choice.

- Review your advance directive to make sure your wishes are still current.

- Have more conversations with your loved ones about your end-of-life wishes.

Things to Do *at Least* Annually

- Make sure a loved one has your passwords and other login information for your phone, your bills, and your online life.

- Adjust how much time and focus you devote to work, close relationships, religion, service to others, self-improvement, physical pleasures, entertainment and travel, and acquiring stuff, to ensure that you're still making the best use of your 119 weekly hours.

- Reassess how well your actions are measuring up to the values that you've chosen to guide your lives as a couple and a family.

Things to Do *at Least* Monthly

- Go on a date with your significant other.
- Volunteer in your community.
- Spend time with someone who's old.
- Work on issues that are causing you regret or guilt.

Things to Do *at Least* Weekly

- Talk for 30 minutes with someone you love, without distraction.

Things to Do Regularly

- Tell relevant, interesting stories to connect the coming generations in your family with their ancestors.
- Contribute to shared medical decisions with your healthcare provider.
- Look to the wise, knowledgeable people around you for help in your pursuit of your mission, meaning, or happiness.
- Remember that it is our nature to grow old, grow sick, and die, and that someday we will be separated from that which we hold dear. This is not a cause for sadness, but a reminder to live well.
- As losses occur in your life, practice coping with them well.
- Reassess the things that fuel your meaning and happiness. Are you enjoying a good balance of both?
- Review your medications with your doctor to ensure they're meeting your needs.
- Resolve family conflicts and estrangements with your loved ones.

Things to Do Every Day

- Appreciate something beautiful, and remember that it's temporary.
- Make the most of your time with your loved ones while you have it.
- Set a good example for the people around you.
- Challenge yourself with a puzzle; a different type of book or magazine than you'd normally read; a documentary about an unfamiliar subject; a new skill; or even a college course.
- Practice eating a healthy diet, exercising, and other healthy lifestyle habits.
- Continue to strive to maintain a flexible, positive attitude.
- Put away your phone and do something interesting for 30 minutes.
- If something is worth doing, do it now. Don't put it off for another day.
- Send out good ripples into your surroundings.
- Double-check your thoughts and actions to make sure you aren't running on autopilot.

And finally, while you're living, never stop being *alive!*

REFERENCES

Introduction

1. Lori Tragesser, interviewed by author, June 2016.

2. "Breast Cancer Statistics," Susan G. Komen, accessed Sept. 13, 2016, http://ww5.komen.org/BreastCancer/Statistics.html.

3. "Breast Cancer Risk in American Women," National Cancer Institute, accessed Sept. 13, 2016, http://www.cancer.gov/types/breast/risk-fact-sheet.

4. "What Are the Key Statistics about Breast Cancer in Men?" American Cancer Society, accessed Sept. 13, 2016, http://www.cancer.org/cancer/breastcancerinmen /detailedguide/breast-cancer-in-men-key-statistics.

5. "Thanks for the Mammories," accessed Sept. 13, 2016, http://loritrag.blogspot.com/.

6. "Living with Stage 4," Fred Hutch, accessed Sept. 13, 2016, https://www.fredhutch .org/en/news/center-news/2014/10/stage-4-metastatic-misunderstood-breast -cancer.html.

7. S. Bayraktar, "Surviving Metastatic Breast Cancer for 18 Years: A Case Report and Review of the Literature," *Breast Journal* 17, no. 5 (2011): 521–24.

8. "Deaths: Final Data for 2013," National Vital Statistics Reports, accessed Sept. 13, 2016, http://www.cdc.gov/nchs/data/nvsr/nvsr64/nvsr64_02.pdf.

9. "Life Tables for the United States Social Security Area 1900–2100," Social Security Administration, accessed Sept. 13, 2016, https://www.ssa.gov/oact/NOTES /pdf_studies/study120.pdf.

10. "New Research Sheds Light on Daily Ad Exposures," SJ Insights, accessed Sept. 13, 2016, https://sjinsights.net/2014/09/29/new-research-sheds-light-on-daily-ad-exposures/.

11. Author interview with Dan Moseley, June 9, 2016.

12. "Traffic Safety Facts," National Highway Traffic Safety Administration, accessed Sept. 13, 2016, https://crashstats.nhtsa.dot.gov/Api/Public/ViewPublication/812124.

Chapter 1

1. Marilyn J. Field and Christine K. Cassel, eds., *Approaching Death: Improving Care at the End of Life* (Washington, DC: National Academy Press, 1997) 29.

2. Scott Murray, "Illness Trajectories and Palliative Care," *BMJ* 330, no. 7498 (2005): 1007–11.

3. Author interview with Suelin Chen, July 7, 2016.

4. Lauren van Scoy, "Can Playing an End-of-Life Conversation Game Motivate People to Engage in Advance Care Planning?" *American Journal of Hospice & Palliative Medicine*, published online July 12, 2016.

5. Author interview with Harriet Warshaw, June 23, 2016.

6. Young Adult, *New York Times,* accessed Sept. 15, 2016, http://www.nytimes.com /books/best-sellers/young-adult/?_r=0.

7. "'Fault in Our Stars' Box Office to Cross $300M Worldwide on Modest Budget: How'd It Happen?" Deadline Hollywood, http://deadline.com/2014/09/fault-in-our -stars-box-office-crosses-300-million-836307/.

8. "Caleb Wilde," Twitter, accessed Sept. 15, 2016, https://twitter.com/calebwilde ?lang=en.

9. "What is Death Cafe?" Death Cafe, accessed Sept. 15, 2016, http://deathcafe.com/what/.

10. "Views on End-of-Life Medical Treatments," Pew Research Center, accessed Sept. 15, 2016, http://www.pewforum.org/2013/11/21/views-on-end-of-life -medical-treatments/.

11. "1-in-4 Older Adults Has Not Discussed Advance Care Planning," Newswise, accessed Nov. 5, 2016, http://www.newswise.com/articles/view/663792/?sc=dwhr &xy=5006852.

12. "Advance Directives," MedlinePlus, accessed Sept. 15, 2016, https://medlineplus .gov/advancedirectives.html.

13. J. J. You, "Barriers to Goals of Care Discussions with Seriously Ill Hospitalized Patients and Their Families: A Multicenter Survey of Clinicians," *JAMA Internal Medicine* 175, no. 4 (2015): 549–56.

14. National Vital Statistics Reports, "United States Life Tables, 2011," accessed Sept. 15, 2016, http://www.cdc.gov/nchs/data/nvsr/nvsr64/nvsr64_11.pdf.

15. "Solving the Mystery Flu That Killed 50 Million People," Time, accessed Sept. 15, 2016, http://time.com/79209/solving-the-mystery-flu-that-killed-50-million-people/.

16. "Mortality and Cause of Death, 1900 vs 2010," UNC Carolina Population Center, accessed Sept. 15, 2016, http://demography.cpc.unc.edu/wp-content/uploads/2014 /06/ID-Mortality-1900-v-2010-e1402580332746.png

17. Marilyn J. Field and Christine K. Cassel, eds., *Approaching Death: Improving Care at the End of Life* (Washington, DC: National Academy Press, 1997) 33.

18. "Health, United States, 2015," Centers for Disease Control and Prevention, accessed Sept. 15, 2016, http://www.cdc.gov/nchs/data/hus/hus15.pdf#019.

19. Harry Sultz, *Health Care USA* (Burlington: Jones & Bartlett Learning, 2010), 75.

20. "*QuickStats*: Percentage Distribution of Deaths, by Place of Death—United States, 2000–2014," Centers for Disease Control and Prevention, accessed Sept. 15, 2016,

http://www.cdc.gov/mmwr/volumes/65/wr/mm6513a6.htm#.

21. "Cutting the High Cost of End-of-Life Care," Time, accessed Sept. 15, 2016, http://time
.com/money/2793643/cutting-the-high-cost-of-end-of-life-care/.

22. "*QuickStats*: Percentage Distribution of Deaths, by Place of Death—United States,
2000–2014," Centers for Disease Control and Prevention, accessed Sept. 15, 2016,
http://www.cdc.gov/mmwr/volumes/65/wr/mm6513a6.htm#.

23. "Patients Served by Hospice in the US: 1982 to 2014," National Hospice and Palliative Care Organization, accessed Sept. 15, 2016, http://www.nhpco.org/sites/default
/files/public/Statistics_Research/Patients_Served.pdf.

24. "America's Care of Serious Illness," Center to Advance Palliative Care, accessed
Sept. 15, https://reportcard.capc.org/wp-content/uploads/2015/08/CAPC-Report
-Card-2015.pdf.

25. "Hospice Care," National Hospice and Palliative Care Organization, page 7,
accessed Sept. 15, 2016, http://www.nhpco.org/about/hospice-care.

26. Stephen J. Connor, "Comparing Hospice and Nonhospice Patient Survival among
Patients Who Die within a Three-Year Window," *Journal of Pain and Symptom
Management* 33, no. 3 (2007): 238–46.

27. Sheldon Solomon, Jeff Greenberg, and Tom Pyszczynski, *The Worm at the Core*
(New York: Random House, 2015).

28. Author interview with Meredith MacMartin, June 8, 2016.

29. Holly McGregor, "Terror Management and Aggression: Evidence That Mortality
Salience Motivates Aggression against Worldview-Threatening Others," *Journal of
Personality and Social Psychology* 74, no. 3 (1998): 590–605.

30. C. R. Cox, "How Sweet It Is to Be Loved by You: The Role of Perceived Regard
in the Terror Management of Close Relationships," *Journal of Personality and Social
Psychology* 102, no. 3 (2012): 616–32.

31. Ilan Dar-Nimrod, "Viewing Death on Television Increases the Appeal of Advertised Products," *Journal of Social Psychology* 152, no. 2 (2012): 199–211.

32. Tomasz Zaleskiewicz, "Saving Can Save from Death Anxiety: Mortality Salience
and Financial Decision-Making," *PLoS One* 2013; 8(11): e79407.

33. JF Bassett, "Terror Management and Reactions to Undocumented Immigrants:
Mortality Salience Increases Aversion to Culturally Dissimilar Others," *Journal of
Social Psychology* 151, no. 2 (2011): 117–20.

34. Crystal Hoyt, "Taking a Turn toward the Masculine: The Impact of Mortality
Salience on Implicit Leadership Theories," *Basic and Applied Social Psychology* 33,
no. 4 (2011): 374–81.

35. Amanda Vicary, "Mortality Salience and Namesaking: Does Thinking about Death

Make People Want to Name Their Children after Themselves?" *Journal of Research in Personality* 45, no. 1 (2011): 138–41.

36. Kenneth Vail, "An Appreciative View of the Brighter Side of Terror Management Processes," *Social Sciences* 4, no. 4 (2015): 1020–45.

37. Author interview with Lisa Iverach, June 13, 2016.

Chapter 2

1. Justin Heckert, "The Hazards of Growing Up Painlessly, *New York Times*, accessed Sept. 16, 2016, http://www.nytimes.com/2012/11/18/magazine/ashlyn-blocker-feels -no-pain.html?_r=0.

2. Yasuhiro Indo, "Congenital Insensitivity to Pain with Anhidrosis," *GeneReviews*. https://www.ncbi.nlm.nih.gov/books/NBK1769/

3. Irvin Yalom, *Staring at the Sun* (San Francisco: Jossey-Bass, 2008) 5–6.

4. Author interview with Victor Strecher, 2016.

5. Jorge Luis Borges, *Collected Fictions* (New York: Penguin Books, 1999) 183–95.

6. Author interview with David Zuniga, June 7, 2016.

7. S. Agras, "The Epidemiology of Common Fears and Phobia," *Comprehensive Psychiatry* 10 (1969): 151–56.

8. Russell Noyes, "Illness Fears in the General Population," *Psychosomatic Medicine* 62 (2000): 318–25.

9. Patricia Furer, "Death Anxiety: A Cognitive-Behavioral Approach," *Journal of Cognitive Psychotherapy* 22, no. 2 (2008): 167–82.

10. "Epicurus," Internet Encyclopedia of Philosophy, accessed Sept. 16, 2016, http://www.iep.utm.edu/epicur/.

11. "Universe Older Than Previously Thought," NASA, accessed Sept. 16, 2016, https://science.nasa.gov/science-news/science-at-nasa/2013/21mar_cmb/.

12. Author interview with William Stephens, Aug. 19, 2016.

13. "Deaths and Mortality," Centers for Disease Control and Prevention, accessed Sept. 16, 2016, http://www.cdc.gov/nchs/fastats/deaths.htm.

14. Author interview with Nicholas Carleton, July 29, 2016.

15. "Statistics," NFDA, accessed Sept. 16, 2016, http://www.nfda.org/news/statistics.

16. "Capsula Mundi," Capsula Mundi, accessed Sept. 16, 2016, http://www.capsulamundi.it/en/.

17. Author interview with Kerry Egan, Aug. 9, 2016.

18. Author interview with Alex Lickerman, June 3, 2016.

19. Alex Lickerman, *The Undefeated Mind: On the Science of Constructing an Indestructible Self* (Deerfield Beach, FL: HCI Books, 2012) 227–29.

20. "Organ Donation Statistics," https://www.organdonor.gov, accessed Sept. 16, 2016, http://www.organdonor.gov/statistics-stories/statistics.html#morestats.

21. "Facts: Did You Know?" American Transplant Foundation, accessed Sept. 16, 2016, http://www.americantransplantfoundation.org/about-transplant/facts-and-myths/.

22. Joshua Newton, "How Does the General Public View Posthumous Organ Donation? A Meta-Synthesis of the Qualitative Literature," *BMC Public Health* 11 (2011).

23. A. Ralph, "Family Perspectives on Deceased Organ Donation," *American Journal of Transplantation* 14 (2014): 923–25.

24. Alexander Batthyany and Pninit Russo-Netzer, eds., *Meaning in Positive and Existential Psychology* (New York: Springer, 2014) 125–37.

25. Stephen R. Harding, "The Influence of Religion on Death Anxiety and Death Acceptance," *Mental Health, Religion & Culture* 8, no. 4 (2005). 253–61

26. Paul Wink, "Does Religiousness Buffer Against the Fear of Death and Dying in Late Adulthood? Findings from a Longitudinal Study," *Journals of Gerontology Series B* 60, no. 4 (2005): 207–14.

27. Lee Ellis, "Religiosity and Fear of Death: A Three-Nation Comparison," *Mental Health, Religion & Culture* 16, no. 2 (2013): 179–99.

Chapter 3

1. Viktor Frankl, *Man's Search for Meaning* (Boston: Beacon Press, 1993).

2. "Man's Search for Meaning," Beacon Press, accessed Sept. 6, 2016, http://www.beacon.org/Mans-Search-for-Meaning-P607.aspx.

3. R. Cohen, "Purpose in Life and Its Relationship to All-Cause Mortality and Cardiovascular Events: A Meta-Analysis," *Psychosomatic Medicine* 78, no. 2 (2016): 122–23.

4. Jessie Dezutter, "Meaning in Life: An Important Factor for the Psychological Well-Being of Chronically Ill Patients?" *Rehabilitation Psychology* 58, no. 4 (2013): 334–41.

5. Patrick L. Hill, "Purpose in Life as a Predictor of Mortality across Adulthood," *Psychological Science* 25, no. 7 (2014): 1482–6.

6. "Michael Steger: What Makes Life Meaningful?" YouTube, accessed Sept. 6, 2016, https://www.youtube.com/watch?v=RLFVoEF2RI0.

7. Michael Steger, interviewed by author, Aug. 3, 2016.

8. "Compassion and the Individual," His Holiness the 14th Dalai Lama of Tibet, accessed Sept. 6, 2016, http://www.dalailama.com/messages/compassion.

9. Roy F. Baumeister, "Some Key Differences between a Happy Life and a Meaningful Life," *Journal of Positive Psychology* 8, no. 6 (2013).

10. Victor J. Strecher, *Life on Purpose* (New York: HarperOne, 2016).

11. Barbara L. Fredrickson, "A Functional Genomic Perspective on Human Well-Being," *PNAS* 110, no. 33 (2013): 13684–89.

12. Samantha J. Heintzelman, "Life Is Pretty Meaningful," *American Psychologist* 69, no. 6 (2014): 561–74.

13. "Mean Age of Mothers Is on Rise: United States, 2000–2014," Centers for Disease Control and Prevention, accessed Sept. 6, 2016, http://www.cdc.gov/nchs/products /databriefs/db232.htm.

14. "Figure FM-3: Average Number of Own Children per Family," US Census Bureau, accessed Sept. 6, 2016, https://www.census.gov/hhes/families/files/graphics/FM-3.pdf.

15. "Google Company," Google, accessed Sept. 7, 2016, https://www.google.com/about /company/.

16. "About Tesla," Tesla, accessed Sept. 7, 2016, https://www.tesla.com/about.

17. Andrew Khouri and Samantha Masunaga, "Tesla's Elon Musk and His Big Ideas: A Brief History," *Los Angeles Times,* May 1, 2015, accessed Sept. 7, 2016, http://www .latimes.com/la-fi-hy-elon-musk-big-ideas-story-so-far-20150501-htmlstory.html.

18. "Mayo Clinic Mission and Values," Mayo Clinic, accessed Sept. 7, 2016, http://www.mayoclinic.org/about-mayo-clinic/mission-values.

19. "About Us," Goodwill Industries International, Inc., accessed Dec. 21, 2016, http://www.goodwill.org/about-us/.

20. Alex Lickerman, *The Undefeated Mind: On the Science of Constructing an Indestructible Self* (Deerfield Beach FL: HCI Books, 2012).

21. Author interview with David Zuniga, June 7, 2016.
Chapter 4

1. Author interview with Bryan Dik, interviewed by author, June 14, 2016.

2. Bryan Dik and Ryan Duffy, *Make Your Job a Calling* (West Conshohocken, PA: Templeton Press, 2013), 45.

3. "Men's Soccer," NCAA, accessed Sept. 13, 2016, http://www.ncaa.org/about /resources/research/mens-soccer.

4. Author interview with Alexandra Solomon, Sept. 1, 2016.

5. Author interview with Susan Newman, Aug. 16, 2016.

6. "US Public Becoming Less Religious," Pew Research Center, accessed Sept. 12, 2016, http://www.pewforum.org/2015/11/03/u-s-public-becoming-less-religious/.

7. "America's Changing Religious Landscape," Pew Research Center, accessed Sept. 12, 2016, http://www.pewforum.org/2015/05/12/americas-changing-religious -landscape/.

8. Author interview with Daryl Van Tongeren, June 20, 2016.

9. Daryl Van Tongeren, "Forgiveness Increases Meaning in Life," *Social Psychological and Personality Science* 6, no. 1 (2015): 47–55, http://spp.sagepub.com/content/6/1 /47.full.pdf+html.

10. Daryl Van Tongeren, "Prosociality Enhances Meaning in Life," *Journal of Positive Psychology* 11, no. 3 (2015): 1–12, https://www.researchgate.net

240 REFERENCES

/publication/277950335_Prosociality_enhances_meaning_in_life.

11. Adam B. Cohen, "The Relation between Religion and Well-Being," *Applied Research in Quality of Life* (2016): 1–15.

12. Author interview with Sara Konrath, Aug. 3, 2016.

13. Daryl Van Tongeren, "Prosociality Enhances Meaning in Life," *Journal of Positive Psychology* 11, no. 3 (2015): 1–12, https://www.researchgate.net/publication /277950335_Prosociality_enhances_meaning_in_life.

14. Morris Okun, "Volunteering by Older Adults and Risk of Mortality: A Meta-Analysis," *Psychology and Aging* 28, no. 2 (2013): 564–77.

15. Sara Konrath, "Motives for Volunteering Are Associated with Mortality Risk in Older Adults," *Health Psychology* 31, no. 1 (2012): 87–96.

16. Helen Y. Weng, "Compassion Training Alters Altruism and Neural Responses to Suffering," *Psychological Science* 24, no. 7 (2013): 1171–80.

17. "Compassion Training," Center for Healthy Minds, accessed Sept. 21, 2016, http://centerhealthyminds.org/well-being-tools/compassion-training/.

18. Constance Furey, *Erasmus, Contarini, and the Religious Republic of Letters* (Cambridge: Cambridge University Press, 2005), 45.

19. "Desiderius Erasmus," Stanford Encyclopedia of Philosophy, accessed Sept. 21, 2016, http://plato.stanford.edu/entries/erasmus/.

20. M. E. Lenehan, "Sending Your Grandparents to University Increases Cognitive Reserve: The Tasmanian Healthy Brain Project," *Neuropsychology* 30, no. 5 (2016): 525–31, http://www.ncbi.nlm.nih.gov/pubmed/26569028.

21. Yaakov Stern, "Cognitive Reserve in Ageing and Alzheimer's Disease," *Lancet Neurology* 11, no. 11 (2012): 1006–12, http://www.ncbi.nlm.nih.gov/pmc/articles /PMC3507991/.

22. Prashanthi Vemuri, "Association of Lifetime Intellectual Enrichment with Cognitive Decline in the Older Population," *JAMA Neurology* 71, no. 8 (2014): 1017–24, http://archneur.jamanetwork.com/article.aspx?articleid=1883334.

23. "The Food Guide Pyramid," United States Department of Agriculture, accessed Sept. 21, 2016, http://www.cnpp.usda.gov/FGP.

Chapter 5

1. "Why Does Time Fly As We Get Older?" Scientific American, accessed Oct. 21, 2016, http://blogs.scientificamerican.com/mind-guest-blog/why-does-time-fly-as-we-get -older/.

2. Author interview with Everett Worthington, July 26, 2016.

3. "The Forgiveness Boost," The Atlantic, accessed Oct. 21, 2016, http://www.the atlantic.com/health/archive/2015/01/the-forgiveness-boost/384796/.

4. Loren Toussaint, "Effects of Lifetime Stress Exposure on Mental and Physical Health in Young Adulthood: How Stress Degrades and Forgiveness Protects Health," *Journal of Health Psychology* 21, no. 6 (2016): 1004–14.

5. S. Akhtar, "Forgiveness Therapy for the Promotion of Mental Well-Being: A Systematic Review and Meta-Analysis," *Trauma, Violence & Abuse* (2016): page ii.

6. J. J. Exline, "Forgiveness, Depressive Symptoms, and Communication at the End of Life: A Study with Family Members of Hospice Patients," *Journal of Palliative Medicine* 15, no. 10 (2012): 1113–19.

7. Barbara L. Fredrickson, "The Broaden-and-Build Theory of Positive Emotions," *Philosophical Transactions of the Royal Society B* (2004): 1367–77.

8. Barbara L. Fredrickson, "The Role of Positive Emotions in Positive Psychology," *American Psychologist* 56, no. 3 (2001): 218–26.

9. "What Is Forgiveness?" Greater Good Science Center, accessed Oct. 21, 2016, http://greatergood.berkeley.edu/topic/forgiveness/definition.

10. Everett L. Worthington, "Forgiveness, Health, and Well-Being: A Review of Evidence for Emotional versus Decisional Forgiveness, Dispositional Forgivingness, and Reduced Unforgiveness," *Journal of Behavioral Medicine* 30, no. 4 (2007): 291–302.

11. "How to REACH Emotional Self-Forgiveness," American Association of Christian Counselors, accessed Sept. 7, 2016, http://www.aacc.net/2013/06/25/how-to-reach-emotional-self-forgiveness/.

12. "What Is Mindfulness?" Greater Good Science Center, accessed Oct. 21, 2016, http://greatergood.berkeley.edu/topic/mindfulness/definition.

13. Author interview with Julie Chippendale, June 8, 2016.

14. Author interview with Nicholas Carleton, July 29, 2016.

15. R. Nicholas Carleton, "Increasingly Certain about Uncertainty: Intolerance of Uncertainty across Anxiety and Depression," *Journal of Anxiety Disorders* 26 (2012): 468–79.

16. R. Nicholas Carleton, "Fearing the Unknown: A Short Version of the Intolerance of Uncertainty Scale," *Journal of Anxiety Disorders* 21 (2007): 105–17.

17. R. Nicholas Carleton, "Increasingly Certain about Uncertainty: Intolerance of Uncertainty across Anxiety and Depression," *Journal of Anxiety Disorders* 26 (2012): 468–79.

18. James F. Boswell, "Intolerance of Uncertainty: A Common Factor in the Treatment of Emotional Disorders," *Journal of Clinical Psychology* 69, no. 6 (2013): 630–45.

19. "Psychotherapy," National Alliance on Mental Illness, accessed Oct. 21, 2016, http://www.nami.org/Learn-More/Treatment/Psychotherapy.

Chapter 6

1. Author interview with Elizabeth Eckstrom, Aug. 11, 2016.

2. Dana E. King, "The Status of Baby Boomers' Health in the United States: The Healthiest Generation?" *JAMA Internal Medicine* 173, no. 5 (2013): 385–86.

3. Dana E. King, "Intake of Key Chronic Disease–Related Nutrients among Baby Boomers," *Southern Medical Journal* 107, no. 6 (2014): 342–47.

4. Aimee Swartz, "James Fries: Healthy Aging Pioneer," *American Journal of Public Health* 98, no. 7 (2008): 1163–66.

5. James F. Fries, "Compression of Morbidity 1980–2011: A Focused Review of Paradigms and Progress," *Journal of Aging Research* (2011). doi: 10.4061/2011/261702

6. Severine Sabia, "Influence of Individual and Combined Healthy Behaviours on Successful Aging," *CMAJ* 184, no. 18 (2012): 1985–92.

7. "Adopt a Mediterranean Diet Now for Better Health Later," Harvard Health Publications, accessed Oct. 21, 2016, http://www.health.harvard.edu/blog/adopt-a-mediterranean-diet-now-for-better-health-later-201311066846.

8. Marta Crous-Bou, "Mediterranean Diet and Telomere Length in Nurses' Health Study: Population Based Cohort Study," *BMJ* 2, no. 349 (2014). doi: 10.1136/bmj.g6674

9. Huaqing Zheng, "Body Mass Index and Risk of Knee Osteoarthritis: Systematic Review and Meta-Analysis of Prospective Studies," *BMJ Open* 2015;5(12). doi:10.1136/bmjopen-2014-007568

10. "Osteoarthritis Symptoms," Arthritis Foundation, accessed Oct. 21, 2016, http://www.arthritis.org/about-arthritis/types/osteoarthritis/symptoms.php.

11. Wojtek Chodzo-Zajko, "Exercise and Physical Activity for Adults," *Medicine & Science in Sports & Exercise* 41, no. 7 (2009): 1510–30.

12. "Alcohol," World Health Organization, accessed Oct. 21, 2016, http://www.who.int/mediacentre/factsheets/fs349/en/.

13. Michael J. Barry, "Shared Decision Making—The Pinnacle of Patient-Centered Care," *New England Journal of Medicine* 366 (2012): 780–81.

14. "Hip Osteoarthritis: Treatment Options," Patient, accessed Oct. 21, 2016, http://patient.info/decision-aids/hip-osteoarthritis-treatment-options.

15. "More Men with Early Prostate Cancer Are Choosing to Avoid Treatment," New York Times, accessed Oct. 21, 2016, http://www.nytimes.com/2016/05/25/health/prostate-cancer-active-surveillance-surgery-radiation.html?_r=0.

16. "Health, United States, 2015," Centers for Disease Control and Prevention, accessed Oct. 21, 2016, http://www.cdc.gov/nchs/data/hus/hus15.pdf.

17. "Merck Manual Professional Version," accessed Oct. 21, 2016, http://www.merckmanuals.com/professional/geriatrics/approach-to-the-geriatric-patient/physical-changes-with-aging.

18. "Multiple Chronic Conditions among Adults Aged 45 and Over: Trends over the Past 10 Years," Centers for Disease Control and Prevention, accessed Oct. 21, 2016, http://www.cdc.gov/nchs/products/databriefs/db100.htm.

19. Author interview with Kathryn Betts Adams, July 28, 2016.

20. J. E. Owens, "Stories of Growth and Wisdom: A Mixed-Methods Study of People Living Well with Pain," *Global Advances in Health and Medicine* 5, no. 1 (2016): 16–28.

21. Lars Tornstam, "Maturing into Gerotranscendence," *Journal of TransPersonal Psychology* 43, no. 2 (2011): 166–80.

22. "Mourning and Reinvention in Mid-Life," Psychology Today, accessed Oct. 21, 2016, https://www.psychologytoday.com/blog/mid-life-what-crisis/201305/mourning-and-reinvention-in-mid-life.

23. "Looking at Wisdom from Mid-Life," Psychology Today, accessed Oct. 21, 2016, https://www.psychologytoday.com/blog/mid-life-what-crisis/201309/looking-wisdom-mid-life.

Chapter 7

1. Author interview with Kerry Egan, Aug. 9, 2016.

2. Johnny Cox, "Making the Healing Difference: Guilt and Regret," *American Journal of Hospice & Palliative Care* 2009: 26(1),64–65. doi: 10.1177/1049909108324358

3. Author interview with Amy Getter, June 16, 2016.

4. Author interview with Kim Mooney, Aug., 2016.

5. Author interview with Marc Agronin, July 29, 2016.

6. "NHPCO's Facts and Figures," National Hospice and Palliative Care Organization, accessed Sept. 16, 2016, http://www.nhpco.org/sites/default/files/public/Statistics_Research/2015_Facts_Figures.pdf.

7. "Medicare Hospice Conditions of Participation Volunteers and Volunteer Managers," National Hospice and Palliative Care Organization, accessed Sept. 16, 2016, http://www.nhpco.org/sites/default/files/public/regulatory/vol_tip%20sheet-Rev%202009.pdf.

8. "Become a Volunteer," Hospice Foundation of America, accessed Oct. 22, 2016, https://hospicefoundation.org/Volunteer.

9. "'Will You Stay with Me?': The No One Dies Alone Program," Modern Medicine Network, accessed Sept. 16, 2016, http://www.modernmedicine.com/modern-medicine/news/modernmedicine/modern-medicine-feature-articles/will-you-stay-me-no-one-dies-al?page=full.

10. S. Claxton-Oldfield, "Hospice Palliative Care Volunteers: The Benefits for Patients, Family Caregivers, and the Volunteers," *Palliative & Supportive Care* 13, no. 3 (2015): 809–13.

244   REFERENCES

11. S. Claxton-Oldfield, "The Impact of Volunteering in Hospice Palliative Care," *American Journal of Hospice & Palliative Care* 24, no. 4 (2007): 259–63.

12. "Selected Long-Term Care Statistics," Family Caregiver Alliance, retrieved Sept. 16, 2016, https://www.caregiver.org/selected-long-term-care-statistics.

13. Eve H. Davison, "Late-Life Emergence of Early-Life Trauma," *Research on Aging* 28, no. 1 (2006): 84–114.

14. "Seinfeld—'The Old Man,'" YouTube, accessed Sept. 16, 2016, https://www.youtube.com/watch?v=fvEYgR9vr6U.

15. Author interview with Nicholas Carleton, July 29, 2016.

16. Search for term "greatest regret" on Legacy.com, Aug. 2016.

17. Author interview with Joshua Coleman, Aug. 15, 2016.

Chapter 8

1. "Jefferson Building Ground Floor," Library of Congress, accessed Sept. 17, 2016, https://www.loc.gov/visit/maps-and-floor-plans/jefferson-building-ground-floor/.

2. StoryCorps, accessed Sept. 17, 2016, https://storycorps.org/.

3. "About," StoryCorps, accessed Sept. 17, 2016, https://storycorps.org/about/.

4. "Frequently Asked Questions," StoryCorps, accessed Sept. 17, 2016, https://storycorps.org/faq/#Bring&Prepare.

5. "Tom Woods and Candace Desmond-Woods," accessed Sept. 17, 2016, https://storycorps.org/listen/tom-woods-and-candace-desmond-woods.

6. "Savannah Phelan and Kellie Phelan," StoryCorps, accessed Sept. 17, 2016, https://storycorps.org/listen/savannah-phelan-and-kellie-phelan.

7. "Priya Morganstern, Ken Morganstern, and Bhavani Jaroff," StoryCorps, accessed Sept. 17, 2016, https://storycorps.org/listen/ken-morganstern-priya-morganstern-and-bhavani-jaroff/.

8. Author interview with Dena Huisman, Aug. 17, 2016.

9. "Legacy," Merriam-Webster, accessed Sept. 17, 2017, http://www.merriam-webster.com/dictionary/legacy.

10. Author interview with Barbara Shaiman, June 17, 2016.

11. "Spielberg Wins at Last with 7 Oscars for 'Schindler's List,'" *New York Times*, accessed Sept. 17, 2016, http://www.nytimes.com/1994/03/22/movies/spielberg-wins-at-last-with-7-oscars-for-schindler-s-list.html.

12. Dena Huisman, "Telling a Family Culture: Storytelling, Family Identity, and Cultural Membership," *Interpersona* 8, no. 2 (2014): 144–58.

13. Author interview with Jo Kline Cebuhar, Aug. 18, 2016.

14. "Randy Pausch, 47, Dies; His 'Last Lecture' Inspired Many to Live with Wonder,"

New York Times, accessed Sept. 17, 2016, http://www.nytimes.com/2008/07/26/us/26pausch.html?_r=0.

15. "Randy Pausch Last Lecture: Achieving Your Childhood Dreams," YouTube, accessed Sept. 17, 2016, https://www.youtube.com/watch?v=ji5_MqicxSo.

16. Author interview with Denise Levenick, Aug. 16, 2016.

Chapter 9

1. Author interview with Patti Anewalt, Aug. 5, 2016.

2. "Timeline—Flight 93, September 11, 2011," National Park Service, accessed Sept. 19, 2016, https://www.nps.gov/flni/learn/historyculture/upload/Timeline_flight_93.pdf.

3. "Good Grief," University of Memphis Magazine, accessed Sept. 19, 2016, https://www.memphis.edu/magazinearchive/v20i3/feat5.html.

4. "Grief, Bereavement, and Coping with Loss," PubMed Health, accessed Oct. 4, 2016, https://www.ncbi.nlm.nih.gov/pubmedhealth/PMH0032576/.

5. Author interview with Elizabeth Horn, Sept. 27, 2016.

6. Thomas Attig, *How We Grieve: Relearning the World* (New York: Oxford University Press, 2011).

7. Sidney Zisook, "Grief and Bereavement: What Psychiatrists Need to Know," *World Psychiatry* 8, no. 2 (2009): 67–74.

8. "Grief, Bereavement, and Coping with Loss," PubMed Health, accessed Oct. 4, 2016, https://www.ncbi.nlm.nih.gov/pubmedhealth/PMH0032576/.

9. M. Katherine Shear, "Complicated Grief," *New England Journal of Medicine* 372 (2015): 153–60.

10. "Is Broken Heart Syndrome Real?" American Heart Association, accessed Oct. 4, 2016, http://www.heart.org/HEARTORG/Conditions/More/Cardiomyopathy/Is-Broken-Heart-Syndrome-Real_UCM_448547_Article.jsp#.V-BYjPkrKUk.

11. Robert A. Neimeyer, "A Social Constructionist Account of Grief: Loss and the Narration of Meaning," *Death Studies* 38, no. 6–10 (2014): 485–98.

12. "John Walsh: 5 Things to Know about the Fugitive Hunter," CNN, accessed Oct. 4, 2016, http://www.cnn.com/2014/07/29/justice/john-walsh-five-things/.

13. "'Apostrophe Laws' Named for Kid Victims on the Wane," USA Today, accessed Oct. 4, 2016, http://www.usatoday.com/story/news/nation/2013/06/12/apostrophe-laws-on-the-wane-/2415963/.

14. "Mission Statement," MADD, accessed Dec. 21, 2016, http://www.madd.org/about-us/mission/.

15. Anthony D. Mancini, "Predictors and Parameters of Resilience to Loss: Toward an Individual Differences Model," *Journal of Personality* 77, no. 6 (2009): 1805–31.

16. "Medicare Benefit Policy Manual," Centers for Medicare & Medicaid Services,
246 REFERENCES

accessed Oct. 4, 2016, https://www.cms.gov/Regulations-and-Guidance/Guidance/Manuals/downloads/bp102c09.pdf.

17. "Medicare Hospice Conditions of Participation Bereavement," National Hospice and Palliative Care Organization, accessed Oct. 4, 2016, http://www.nhpco.org/sites/default/files/public/regulatory/Bereavement_tip_sheet.pdf.

18. M. Katherine Shear, "Optimizing Treatment of Complicated Grief," *JAMA Psychiatry* 73, no. 7 (2016): 685–94.

19. Sidney Zisook, "Bereavement: Course, Consequences, and Care," *Current Psychiatry Reports* 16 (2014).

20. "Depression (Major Depressive Disorder)," Mayo Clinic, accessed Oct. 4, 2016, http://www.mayoclinic.org/diseases-conditions/depression/basics/definition/CON-20032977?p=1.

21. "Post-Traumatic Stress Disorder," Mayo Clinic, accessed Oct. 4, 2016, http://www.mayoclinic.org/diseases-conditions/post-traumatic-stress-disorder/basics/symptoms/con-20022540.

Chapter 10

1. "General Statistics," Insurance Institute for Highway Safety/Highway Loss Data Institute, accessed Sept. 17, 2016, http://www.iihs.org/iihs/topics/t/general-statistics/fatalityfacts/gender.

2. Author interview with Chanel Reynolds, June 8, 2016.

3. Author interview with Carolyn Moor, July 14, 2016.

4. "Deaths: Final Data for 2013," Centers for Disease Control and Prevention, accessed Sept. 17, 2016, http://www.cdc.gov/nchs/data/nvsr/nvsr64/nvsr64_02.pdf.

5. "Meet 2 People Whose Emergency Funds Rescued Them," Bankrate, accessed Sept. 18, 2016, http://www.bankrate.com/finance/consumer-index/financial-security-charts-0621.aspx.

6. "Final Stewart Crash Report Released," ABC News, accessed March 7, 2017, http://abcnews.go.com/US/story?id=94839.

Chapter 11

1. Author interview with Betty Kramer, Aug. 25, 2016.

2. Author interview with Simon Oczkowski, Aug. 8, 2016.

3. Author interview with Harriet Warshaw, June 23, 2016.

4. "Your Conversation Starter Kit," The Conversation Project, accessed Sept. 14, 2016, http://theconversationproject.org/starter-kit/intro/.

5. Author interview with Judy Thomas, July 28, 2016.

6. "In Unforgettable Final Act, a King Got Revenge on His Killers," *New York Times*, accessed Sept. 14, 2016, http://www.nytimes.com/2005/01/25/health
REFERENCES   247

/in-unforgettable-final-act-a-king-got-revenge-on-his-killers.html.

7. Atul Gawande, *Being Mortal* (New York: Picador, 2015).

8. "Advance Health Care Directives Frequently Asked Questions for Consumers," Coalition for Compassionate Care of California, accessed Sept. 15, 2016, http://coalitionccc .org/wp-content/uploads/2014/10/AHCD_Frequently_Asked_Questions.pdf.

9. "Download Your State's Advance Directives," CaringInfo, accessed Sept. 15, 2016, http://www.caringinfo.org/i4a/pages/index.cfm?pageid=3289.

10. "Five Wishes," Aging with Dignity, accessed Dec. 22, 2016, https://agingwith dignity.org/docs/default-source/default-document-library/product-samples /fwsample.pdf?sfvrsn=2.

11. Author interview with Lori Tragesser, June 2016.

12. "Indiana Advance Directive—Planning for Important Health Care Decisions," accessed Sept. 15, 2016, http://www.caringinfo.org/files/public/ad/Indiana.pdf.

13. Author interview with Bud Hammes, Sept. 15, 2016.

14. "Giving Someone a Power of Attorney for Your Health Care," American Bar Association, accessed Sept. 16, 2016, http://www.americanbar.org/groups/law_aging/ resources/health_care_decision_making/power_atty_guide_and_form_2011.html.

15. "Advance Health Care Directives Frequently Asked Questions for Consumers," Coalition for Compassionate Care of California, accessed Sept. 16, 2016, http://coalition ccc.org/wp-content/uploads/2014/10/AHCD_Frequently_Asked_Questions.pdf.

16. Author interview with Lauren Van Scoy, July 29, 2016.

17. Barbara Gomes, "Heterogeneity and Changes in Preferences for Dying at Home: A Systematic Review," *BMC Palliative Care* (2013).

18. Y. S. Kim, "The Natural History of Changes in Preferences for Life-Sustaining Treatments and Implications for Inpatient Mortality in Younger and Older Hospitalized Adults," *Journal of the American Geriatric Society* 64, no. 5 (2016): 981–89.

Chapter 12

1. Author interview with Lauren Van Scoy, July 29, 2016.

2. Alexander Smith, "Half of Older Americans Seen in Emergency Department in Last Month of Life; Most Admitted to Hospital, and Many Die There," *Health Affairs* 31, no. 6 (2012): 1277–85.

3. "Trends in Cancer Care Near the End of Life," Dartmouth Institute for Health Policy & Clinical Practice, accessed Sept. 22, 2016, http://www.dartmouthatlas.org /downloads/reports/Cancer_brief_090413.pdf.

4. Derek Angus, "Toward Better ICU Use at the End of Life," *JAMA* 315, no. 3 (2016): 255–56.

5. Author interview with Judy Thomas, July 28, 2016.

6. Author interview with Ferdinando Mirarchi, Aug. 25, 2016.

7. Author interview with Malcolm Mattes, Aug. 18, 2016.

8. Hunter Groninger, "Samuel Beckett's 'Rockaby': Dramatizing the Plight of the Solitary Elderly at Life's End," *Perspectives in Biology and Medicine* 50, no. 2 (2007): 260–75.

9. Author interview with Hunter Groninger, Aug. 18, 2016.

10. Author interview with Simon Oczkowski, Aug. 8, 2016.

11. Author interview with Meredith MacMartin, June 8, 2016.

12. Diane E. Meier, "Teaching Doctors When to Stop Treatment," Washington Post, accessed Sept. 22, 2016, https://www.washingtonpost.com/national/health-science /teaching-doctors-when-to-stop-treatment/2014/05/19/e643d190-caf5-11e3-93eb -6c0037dde2ad_story.html.

13. Monica Krishnan, "Predicting Life Expectancy in Patients with Advanced Incurable Cancer: A Review," *Journal of Supportive Oncology* 11 (2013): 68–74.

14. H. J. Warraich, "Accuracy of Physician Prognosis in Heart Failure and Lung Cancer: Comparison between Physician Estimates and Model Predicted Survival," *Palliative Medicine* 30, no. 7 (2016): 684–89.

15. "Talking with Your Doctor about Prognosis," Cancer.net, accessed Sept. 22, 2016, http://www.cancer.net/blog/2014-08/talking-your-doctor-about-prognosis.

16. Douglas B. White, "Toward Shared Decision Making at the End of Life in Intensive Care Units," *Archives of Internal Medicine* 167 (2007): 461–67.

17. Institute of Medicine, *Dying in America* (Washington: National Academies Press, 2015).

18. E. B. Rubin, "States Worse Than Death among Hospitalized Patients with Serious Illnesses," *JAMA Internal Medicine* 176, no. 10 (2016): 1557–59.

19. "How Doctors Die," Zocalo, accessed Sept. 23, 2016, http://www.zocalopublicsquare .org/2011/11/30/how-doctors-die/ideas/nexus/.

20. Vyjeyanthi S. Periyakoil, "Do Unto Others: Doctors' Personal End-of-Life Resuscitation Preferences and Their Attitudes toward Advance Directives," *PLOS One* 9, no. 5 (2014).

21. Saket Girotra, "Trends in Survival after In-Hospital Cardiac Arrest," *New England Journal of Medicine* 367, no. 20 (2012): 1912–20.

22. Author interview with Judy Thomas, July 28, 2016.

23. Scott Halpern, "Toward Evidence-Based End-of-Life Care," *New England Journal of Medicine* 373 (2015): 2001–3.
Chapter 13

1. Author interview with Karen Wyatt, June 9, 2016.

2. Barbara Gomes, "Heterogeneity and Changes in Preferences for Dying at Home: A Systematic Review," *BMC Palliative Care* 12, no. 7 (2013).
REFERENCES   249

3. Sheri M. Kittelson, "Palliative Care Symptom Management," *Critical Care Nursing Clinics of North America* 27 (2015): 315–39.

4. Mellar P. Davis, "What Is the Difference between Palliative Care and Hospice Care?" *Cleveland Clinic Journal of Medicine* 82, no. 9 (2015): 569–71.

5. Melissa D. Aldridge, "Education, Implementation, and Policy Barriers to Greater Integration of Palliative Care: A Literature Review," *Palliative Medicine* 30, no. 3 (2016): 224–39.

6. Shalini Dalal, "Association between a Name Change from Palliative to Supportive Care and the Timing of Patient Referrals at a Comprehensive Cancer Center," *Oncologist* 16, no. 1 (2011): 105–11.

7. Sheri M. Kittelson, "Palliative Care Symptom Management," *Critical Care Nursing Clinics of North America* 27 (2015): 315–39.

8. Jennifer S. Temel, "Early Palliative Care for Patients with Metastatic Non–Small-Cell Lung Cancer," *New England Journal of Medicine* 363, no. 8 (2010): 733–42.

9. Author interview with Malcolm Mattes, Aug. 18, 2016.

10. Author interview with Meredith MacMartin, June 8, 2016.

11. "Heart Failure Fact Sheet," Centers for Disease Control and Prevention, accessed Sept. 30, 2016, http://www.cdc.gov/dhdsp/data_statistics/fact_sheets/fs_heart_failure.htm.

12. Clyde W. Yancy, "2013 ACCF/AHA Guideline for the Management of Heart Failure," *Circulation* 128 (2013): e240–327.

13. "Palliative Care for Patients with Heart Failure," American College of Cardiology, accessed Sept. 30, 2016, https://www.acc.org/latest-in-cardiology/articles/2016/02/11/08/02/palliative-care-for-patients-with-heart-failure?w_nav=LC.

14. "Classes of Heart Failure," American Heart Association, accessed Sept. 30, 2016, http://www.heart.org/HEARTORG/Conditions/HeartFailure/AboutHeartFailure/Classes-of-Heart-Failure_UCM_306328_Article.jsp#.V-v94fkrKUk.

15. "Implantable Cardioverter Defibrillator (ICD)," American Heart Association, accessed Sept. 30, 2016, http://www.heart.org/HEARTORG/Conditions/Arrhythmia/PreventionTreatmentofArrhythmia/Implantable-Cardioverter-Defibrillator-ICD_UCM_448478_Article.jsp#.V-v_cPkrKUk.

16. Melissa D. Aldridge, "Education, Implementation, and Policy Barriers to Greater Integration of Palliative Care: A Literature Review," *Palliative Medicine* 30, no. 3 (2016): 224–39.

17. C. Scibetta, "The Costs of Waiting: Implications of the Timing of Palliative Care Consultation among a Cohort of Decedents at a Comprehensive Cancer Center," *Journal of Palliative Medicine* 19, no. 1 (2016): 69–75.

18. "Paying for Hospice," National Hospice and Palliative Care Organization, accessed Sept. 30, 2016, http://www.caringinfo.org/i4a/pages/index.cfm?pageid=3358.

250 REFERENCES

19. "Hospice FAQs," National Hospice and Palliative Care Organization, accessed Sept. 30, 2016, http://www.nhpco.org/about-hospice-and-palliative-care/hospice-faqs.

20. Susan L. Vogel, "What Physicians Should Know about Hospice," *Ochsner Journal* 11, no. 4 (2011).

21. "The Hospice Team," National Hospice and Palliative Care Organization, accessed Sept. 30, 2016, http://www.caringinfo.org/i4a/pages/index.cfm?pageid=3357.

22. "Hospice FAQs," National Hospice and Palliative Care Organization, accessed Sept. 30, 2016, http://www.nhpco.org/about-hospice-and-palliative-care/hospice-faqs.

23. David K. Meagher and David E. Balk, eds., *Handbook of Thanatology* (New York: Routledge, 2013).

24. "NHPCO's Facts and Figures—2015 Edition," National Hospice and Palliative Care Organization, accessed Sept. 30, 2016, http://www.nhpco.org/sites/default/files /public/Statistics_Research/2015_Facts_Figures.pdf.

25. Author interview with Hunter Groninger, Aug. 18, 2016.

26. "Serious Illness Conversation Guide," Ariadne Labs, accessed Sept. 30, 2016, https://www.ariadnelabs.org/wp-content/uploads/sites/2/2015/08/Serious-Illness -Conversation-Guide-5.22.15.pdf.

27. Rachelle E. Bernacki, "Communication about Serious Illness Care Goals," *JAMA Internal Medicine* 174, no. 12 (2014): 1994–2003.

28. "How to Talk to Your Doctor," The Conversation Project, accessed Sept. 30, 2016, http://theconversationproject.org/wp-content/uploads/2016/06/TCP-TalkToYourDr -v1.2.pdf.

29. Author interview with Kerry Egan, Aug. 9, 2016.

30. Author interview with Meredith MacMartin, June 8, 2016.

31. Author interview with Amy Getter, June 16, 2016.

32. "Social Workers in Hospice and Palliative Care," National Association of Social Workers, accessed March 7, 2017, http://workforce.socialworkers.org/studies /profiles/Hospice.pdf.

33. Marilyn J. Field and Christine K. Cassel, eds., *Approaching Death: Improving Care at the End of Life* (Washington, DC: National Academy Press, 1997).

34. "The Dying Process," National Hospice and Palliative Care Organization, accessed Sept. 30, 2016, http://www.caringinfo.org/files/public/brochures/Understanding theDyingProces.pdf.

Chapter 14

1. Author interview with Gail Rubin, Sept. 30, 2016.

2. Burden S. Lundgren, "Banishing Death: The Disappearance of the Appreciation of Mortality," *Omega* 61, no.3 (2010): 223–49.

REFERENCES   251

3. Author interview with Josh Slocum, Sept. 27, 2016.

4. "Statistics," National Funeral Directors Association, accessed Nov. 3, 2016, http://www.nfda.org/news/statistics.

5. "Quick Guide to Legal Requirements for Home Funerals in Your State," National Home Funeral Alliance, accessed Nov. 3, 2016, http://homefuneralalliance.org /wp-content/uploads/2016/01/Quick-Guide-to-Home-Funerals-By-State.pdf.

6. Daniel Callahan, "Death, Mourning, and Medical Progress," *Perspectives in Biology and Medicine* 52, no. 1 (2009): 103–15.

7. William G. Hoy, *Do Funerals Matter?* (New York: Routledge, 2013).

INDEX

Clergy member, discussing religion with, 70–71
Cognitive behavioral therapy, 97
Cognitive reserve, education increasing, 75
Coleman, Joshua, 130–33, 131, 132, 133
Community, like-minded
    religion as, 68
    for supporting life's meaning, 50
Compassion
    for self, 92
    for supporting life's meaning, 49
Compassion training, 74
Complicated grief, 156–57, 160–61, 161
Compression of morbidity, 105
Concentration camps, 40–41, 44
Conflicts, family
    preventing, 185–87
    resolving, 233
    sources of, 184–85
Consciousness, transitioning after death, 29
Conversation Project, The, 6–7, 178, 187, 203, 216–17
Conversations about death
    benefits of, xv, xviii–xxi, 173, 178–80
    emergence of, xvii, 5–7
    fear of, 19
    necessity of, 176–77
    questions exploring, 20
Conversations about end-of-life care, avoiding, 8–9
CPR, 8, 196–97, 201
Create the Good and Elder Helpers, 126
Cremation, 32, 225
Critical illness, vs. end of life, 198
Cultural structures
    for managing fear of death, 14–15, 17
    questions exploring, 21

D

Dalai Lama, 43
Death
    accidental, 164–65, 175
    activities readjusting view on
        assuming preparedness for death, 29
        considering promise behind pain, 33
        developing stoic attitude, 27–29

        discovering your life's meaning, 35–36
        distracting yourself from fear of death, 33, 35
        scanning for death anxiety, 25–27
        thinking about time before birth, 27
        thinking about what you leave behind, 30–32
    awareness of
        benefits of, 23
        in humans vs. animals, 14
    belief in life after, 68
    causes of
        modern-day, 10
        most common, 164, 165
        in past, 10, 223–24
    conversations about
        benefits of, xviii–xxi, 173, 178–80
        emergence of, xvii, 5–7
        fear of, 19
        necessity of, 176–77
        questions exploring, 20
    denial of, 25, 35
    family conflict and, 184–87
    fear of
        avoidance for coping with, xvi–xvii, xviii
        exercise for examining, 38–39
        inability to subdue, 23
        managing, 13, 14–15, 17, 26–27, 35, 94–95, 100, 111–12
    "good"
        defining, 177, 232
        factors determining, xiv, 51
        meaning of, 13
        questions exploring, 20
        steps toward, 26 (see also End-of-life planning)
    health states worse than, 197
    messages sent after, 159, 175
    place of
        home, 10, 11, 14, 188, 207, 209, 224, 225
        hospice (see Hospice care)
        hospital, 10, 11, 14, 209, 224
    preparing for, 29, 149
    rating, 38
    religion and, 37, 39
    seniors' acceptance of, 124, 127
    statistics on, 25–26

Death *(cont.)*
  study of, xvii
  sudden, xiv, xv–xvi, xx, 3, **4**, 10, 164–65
    preparing for, 167–74
    preventing, <u>175</u>
  symptoms preceding, 219–20
  as taboo topic, 5
    reasons for, 10–11
  thoughts of, behaviors inspired by,
    15–19
  trajectories of, 3–4, **3**, **4**, 29
Death anxiety. *See* Death, fear of
Deathbed forgiveness, 86
Death Cafe, 7
Decisional forgiveness, 88
Decision making, shared, in healthcare,
  108–9, 195–97, 233
Deliberate living, xiv
Denial of death, 25, 35
Depression
  after death of loved one, 160, 161
  end-of-life, 220
  forgiveness reducing, 86
  major, grief and, <u>161</u>
  mindfulness relieving, 91
  from physical pain, 219
  treatment for, 97
  volunteerism reducing, 72
Dickerson, Bob, <u>107</u>
Diet, Mediterranean, 105–6
Digestive issues, at end of life, 219–20
Dik, Bryan, 59–60, 61, 62–63
Dirty suffering, 92
Disability insurance, 168–69
Distress, working on sources of, 126–30
Divorce, family estrangement from,
  130–31
DNR orders, 201, <u>201</u>, 205
Documentaries, on end-of-life decisions,
  <u>189</u>
Documents. *See also specific documents*
  advance care planning, 201–5
  financial and legal, 169–70, <u>172</u>, <u>173</u>, 188
Doka, Kenneth, 153
Donations, as altruistic act, 72, 73, 74
Do Not Resuscitate (DNR) orders, 201, <u>201</u>,
  205
Doughty, Caitlin, 7
Drinking alcohol, 108
Drug review, 110, 233

Durable power of attorney, 170
Dying people, spending time with, 125–26,
  231

E

Eckstrom, Elizabeth, 103, 104, 105, 106,
  108, 110
Egan, Kerry, 33, 121, 217, <u>221</u>
Elderly people
  discussing death with, 188
  as mentors, 124–26, <u>127</u>
  rising above old age, <u>112</u>
  spending time with, 100, 233
Electronic distractions, 171–72
Emergency room visits, 191
Emergency savings, 169
Emotional changes, at end of life, 220
Emotional forgiveness, 88
End-of-life care
  age-related preferences for, <u>188</u>
  aggressive, drawbacks of, 10–11
  conversations about
    avoiding, 8–9
    with healthcare providers (*see*
      Healthcare providers)
    necessity of, 9, <u>208</u>
  cost of, 11
  doctors' choices for themselves, <u>200</u>
  documentaries on, <u>189</u>
  facing decisions about, 109–10
  family conflicts about, 184–87
  growing control over, 11–12
  in hospice (*see* Hospice care)
  in hospital, 177–78, 190–92
  palliative, 11–12, <u>12</u>, 210–14, 217
  personal growth during, 217–19
  specified in advance directive (*see*
    Advance directive)
  values influencing, 180–81, <u>189</u>
End-of-life conversation game, <u>6</u>
End-of-life lessons, shared in ethical will,
  142
End-of-life planning
  Cake guide to, 5–6
  conversations about, 177–80, 232
    benefits of, xv, 174, 177
  ethical will and, <u>143</u>
  exercises exploring, <u>189</u>

periodic reviews of, 187–88
questions exploring, 20
reducing anxiety about, 26
story about, 30–31
End-of-life symptoms, 219–20
Entertainment, 77, **83**
Epictetus, 28
Epicurus, 27
Erasmus, Desiderius, 75
Estrangement. *See* Family estrangement
Ethical will, 140–43, 143, 175, 177, 231
Eudaimonia, 45
Executor, choosing, 169
Exercise
daily, 234
recommended amount of, 106, 108
story about, 107
Extremis (documentary), 189

F

Falls, 219
Family conflict
preventing, 185–87
resolving, 233
sources of, 184–85
Family estrangement
addressing, in ethical will, 142
causes of, 130–31
resolving, 131–33, 233
Family heirlooms, curating, 144–46, 146,
231
Family identity, revealed in storytelling,
137–38
Family relationships, nurturing, 64–67, 65
Fatigue, as end-of-life symptom, 219
Fault in Our Stars, The, 7
Fear of death
avoidance for coping with, xvi–xvii, xviii
exercise for examining, 38–39
inability to subdue, 23
managing, 13, 14–15, 17, 26–27, 35,
94–95, 100, 111–12
rating, 38
religion and, 37, 39
statistics on, 25–26
Fear of the unknown, 94
Financial discussions, 173
Financial planning, 136, 167–69

Five Wishes, xiv, 181, 203
Flexibility exercises, 108
Flight 93 heroes on September 11,
151–52
Flu pandemic of 1918, 10
Food Guide Pyramid, 76
Forgiveness, 231
benefits of, 69, 86
decisional vs. emotional, 88
at end of life, 218
exercise exploring, 101
"letting it go" vs., 87
meaning of, 87–88
qualities helping with, 90
REACH approach to, 88–89
seeking, in ethical will, 142
of self, 89
story about, 85–86
Frankl, Viktor, 40–41, 44
Fredrickson, Barbara, 87
Friendships, nurturing, 67
Funeral celebrant, 222, 223
Funeral customs, changes in, 32, 224–25
Funeral directing, 224, 225
Funeral planning, 222–28, 229, 232
Furer, Patricia, 26
Future, uncertainty of, 85, 95–96
coping with, 96–100

G

Gawande, Atul, 180, 189, 215
Gee, Elizabeth, 159
Gee, Rebekah, 159
Generosity, for supporting life's meaning,
49
Gerotranscendence, 112
Getter, Amy, 122, 123, 218
Get Your Shit Together Web site, 167
Goals, process vs. outcome, 65
Golden Rule, 92
"Good death"
defining, 177, 232
factors determining, xiv, 51
meaning of, 13
questions exploring, 20
steps toward, 26 (*see also* End-of-life
planning)
Goodwill, mission statement of, 48

M